'*Rethinking Secondary Mental Healthcare: A Perceptual Control Theory Perspective* provides a comprehensive deconstruction of the limitations of current mental healthcare design and delivery. Whilst the critiques in this book are stark, I don't think any of the observations of current provision will be received as a blindside by practitioners. An achievement of the authors is that they have been able to synthesise, using the theoretical lens of Perceptual Control Theory, and write about, their collective experiences as clinicians and users of mental health services, without the undertone of blame or *ressentiment* that often (perhaps, understandably) characterises critiques of psychiatry. This should enable the radical yet practicable ideas and solutions to be confronted without moral injury to any individual or group who have a stake in the quality and safety of mental health services. The deficiencies in care and compassion that are outlined in the book are, after all, a product of systemic rather than individual failings (i.e., conceptualisations of mental distress that are impersonal and of questionable validity, the pervasive experience of being 'too ill' or 'not ill enough' to receive any or certain types of support, and arbitrary limits set on the duration and intensity of the support that is offered). The book's fundamental proposition is that mental service design and delivery should be transformed via radical shifts in the ways that behaviour and distress are conceptualised. Namely, that behaviour is a product of efforts to control perceptual input, distress is a consequence of conflicting goals in the attainment of desired perceptual states, and that effective support should be characterised by the facilitated reorganisation of goal conflicts to reduce distress. It is, fundamentally, a profoundly optimistic text that everyone working in mental health should read.'

Owen Price, *Senior Lecturer in Mental Health Nursing, University of Manchester*

'This text will – I suspect – force professional readers to question many assumptions they hold about the nature of psychological distress and its alleviation, whilst simultaneously striking service users as common sense. Rooted in PCT, the text has wide-ranging implications for the way services are designed and delivered, advocating for the allocation of control to service users wherever possible. Time will tell whether the proposals stand up to empirical testing and deliver on the promise of more effective and efficient care. Irrespective, the over-arching aims of the text are I believe commendable and much needed in the context of over-stretched services.'

Marc Tibber, *Lecturer in Clinical Psychology, University College London*

'A shroud of pessimism has long stymied secondary care mental health services. The people who use them have been viewed as passive recipients of their own care. In this brilliant book, Robert Griffiths and colleagues draw from Perceptual Control Theory to reimagine services that place people as central agents in their own recovery. People are driven by individual goals and are seen as controllers of their own perceptions. Given the right environment, people are capable of solving the inevitable conflicts that emerge when dealing with the complexity of their lives. The challenge then, is to create environments that allow people and families to creatively address these conflicts, in order to find their own solutions. This book provides a blueprint for services to do just that, and in doing so, moves secondary mental health care to a place of hope and optimism.'

James Kelly, *Lecturer in Clinical Psychology, Lancaster University; and Consultant Clinical Psychologist, Greater Manchester Mental NHS Foundation Trust*

'This original and insightful text offers a fresh perspective on the organisation of mental health care and support. The recognition that control over aspects of one's life, or lack of it, might be the most crucial consideration regarding disturbances to mental health is the pivotal touchstone for examining identified shortcomings of mental health services and pointing to solutions. The proposed remedies appear to have great promise in tackling the alienating features of contemporary services, offering a route to more democratic, relational, person-centred responses. Even if the suggested approach to redesign is not to be adopted wholesale, this book offers clear food for thought for practitioners, service users and families who are rightly concerned about the lack of choice within services overly reliant upon coercion rather than consent.'

Mick McKeown, *Professor of Democratic Mental Health, University of Central Lancashire*

'Radical, practical and humane. This work deserves to be a seminal text in the field of secondary mental healthcare and required reading for students, practitioners and managers who wish to be a part of the solution, rather than the problem.'

Nathan Filer, *author of* This Book Will Change Your Mind About Mental Health *and* The Shock of the Fall

'As many mental health services seek to redefine how care is provided, this book gives a theoretically sound framework for coherent patient-perspective-care. Perceptual control theory is offered as a guiding model for mental health services and potentially for shaping communities and society. As a service model and an approach to psychological therapy, PCT gives us something properly new and inviting as an alternative. As a psychological therapy, Method of Levels is truly oriented to patients' priorities, from the timing and duration of sessions to the moment-by-moment content. The book itself is a collaboration between those who have used mental health services and those who work in them. The superb writing in this book is made richer with the views and stories of patients.'

Christopher Whiteley, *Chief Psychologist, Central and North West London NHS Foundation Trust*

'This book succeeds in that all too rare a feat of being both an enjoyable read, alongside explaining some important ideas in easily digestible form. As a clinical psychologist within the NHS who, in addition to delivering psychological therapy, is also involved in service evaluation, design, and management, there are many lessons contained within these pages for me to consider. As a parent of two feisty children, the lessons the book has taught me about control, conflict and reorganisation have also contributed towards me upping my game on the parenting front. So, if you want to improve your standard of therapy, or survive and thrive within services, which we all know have a long way to go, or if you want a solid strategy to remain present and compassionate alongside feisty family or friends of your own, then give yourself the chance to enjoy this book like I did.'

John Mulligan, *Lead Clinical Psychologist,*
Manchester Early Intervention Service,
Greater Manchester Mental Health NHS Foundation Trust

'This is the most important and exciting book I've read in a long time. It explains in everyday language recent developments in psychological science which have profound implications, and the potential completely to transform mental health services. The principles it sets out are revolutionary, but also simple – and liberating for both clinicians and those experiencing mental health problems. The book is supremely practical too, and full of stories that inspire.'

Anne Cooke, *Consultant Clinical Psychologist,*
Clinical Director, Doctoral Programme in Clinical Psychology,
Canterbury Christ Church University

Rethinking Secondary Mental Healthcare

This book considers how principles derived from a theory of human behaviour – Perceptual Control Theory – can be applied to create mental health services that are more effective, efficient, and humane.

Authored by clinicians, academics, and experts-by-experience, the text explores the way Perceptual Control Theory (PCT) principles can be applied within the secondary mental healthcare system – from the overall commissioning and design of services to the practice of individual clinicians. A range of topics relevant to the delivery of secondary mental healthcare are covered, including community and inpatient working, the delivery of individual psychological therapy, the use of restrictive practices, and working with relatives and carers. The book concludes by describing PCT's unique contribution to the field of mental healthcare.

The book, one of the first of its kind, will be of interest to students and practitioners from a range of health and social care backgrounds, as well as service managers, commissioners, academics, and policymakers.

Robert Griffiths is Lecturer in Mental Health at The University of Manchester. He is also Director of the Mental Health Nursing Research Unit based in Greater Manchester NHS Foundation Trust.

Vyv Huddy is Lecturer in Clinical Psychology and Academic Director on the University of Sheffield Doctorate in Clinical Psychology where he provides training, supervision, and mentoring to postgraduate clinical psychologists in training.

Stuart Eaton is an expert-by experience and former registered mental health nurse, and has ten years' experience of working in secondary care mental health services.

Jasmine Waldorf is an expert-by experience, mental health advocate, and community arts practitioner currently leading art workshops for adults with severe mental illness at Arts Network Charity. She is also a mentor for Sydenham Arts, supporting young people in Lewisham who are pursuing careers in the creative industries.

Warren Mansell is Professor of Mental Health at Curtin University, Perth. He has published over 100 peer-reviewed works on Perceptual Control Theory and its application to mental health, including two therapy manuals, and two edited interdisciplinary handbooks.

Rethinking Secondary Mental Healthcare

A Perceptual Control Theory Perspective

Robert Griffiths, Vyv Huddy,
Stuart Eaton, Jasmine Waldorf,
and Warren Mansell

Routledge
Taylor & Francis Group
LONDON AND NEW YORK

Designed cover image: © Image designed by Nicholas Young

First published 2024
by Routledge
4 Park Square, Milton Park, Abingdon, Oxon OX14 4RN

and by Routledge
605 Third Avenue, New York, NY 10158

Routledge is an imprint of the Taylor & Francis Group, an informa business

British Library Cataloguing-in-Publication Data
A catalogue record for this book is available from the British Library

Library of Congress Cataloging-in-Publication Data
Names: Griffiths, Robert (Lecturer in mental health), author. | Huddy, Vyv, author. | Eaton, Stuart, 1973- author. | Waldorf, Jasmine, author. | Mansell, Warren, author.
Title: Rethinking secondary mental healthcare : a perceptual control theory perspective / Robert Griffiths, Vyv Huddy, Stuart Eaton, Jasmine Waldorf, and Warren Mansell.
Description: Abingdon, Oxon ; New York, NY : Routledge, 2024. | Includes bibliographical references and index. |
Identifiers: LCCN 2023022071 (print) | LCCN 2023022072 (ebook) | ISBN 9780367485085 (hbk) | ISBN 9780367485061 (pbk) | ISBN 9781003041344 (ebk)
Subjects: LCSH: Mental health counseling--Methodology. | Perceptual control theory.
Classification: LCC RC466 .G75 2024 (print) | LCC RC466 (ebook) | DDC 362.2072--dc23/eng/20230807
LC record available at https://lccn.loc.gov/2023022071
LC ebook record available at https://lccn.loc.gov/2023022072

ISBN: 978-0-367-48508-5 (hbk)
ISBN: 978-0-367-48506-1 (pbk)
ISBN: 978-1-003-04134-4 (ebk)

DOI: 10.4324/9781003041344

Typeset in Times New Roman
by SPi Technologies India Pvt Ltd (Straive)

Contents

Preface

This is a book about how mental health services can be designed to help people work towards personally meaningful goals. While there was sufficient similarity between our goals as authors to enable us to collaborate in the writing of this book, a key tenet of Perceptual Control Theory (PCT) is that no two people will share an identical set of goals. In the spirit of PCT, therefore, we thought it would be apt for us to start this book by telling you something about the personal motivations of each of the authors for writing it.

Robert Griffiths

The first time I heard the term 'Perceptual Control Theory' (PCT) was in around 2009 while reading an article written by Warren Mansell (Mansell, 2005). I didn't realise at the time that the theory described in the article would have such a profound impact on me, both professionally and personally.

By the time I read Warren's article, I had been working in mental health services for just over a decade. First as a support worker, then as a community mental health nurse, and then, after completing post-qualifying training in cognitive behavioural therapy (CBT), as a psychological therapist. After registering as a mental health nurse in 2002, all of my clinical experience has involved working in community mental health teams – first in Assertive Outreach and then in Early Intervention in Psychosis services.

By 2009, I was becoming interested in approaches to therapy that moved beyond traditional CBT, including 'third-wave' cognitive therapies – Acceptance and Commitment Therapy and Compassion Focused Therapy, for example. It seemed as if all the different approaches to therapy that I was learning about could be helpful for some patients, some of the time. But the more I learned about these different approaches to therapy, the less things seemed to make sense, and the more questions sprang up for me.

When was it appropriate to use therapy X rather than therapy Y, for example? Was it possible to integrate some elements of different therapies, and, if so, how should that integration take place? What about the fact that the various approaches all recommended that therapists engage in such different activities during therapy sessions (e.g., thought diaries, chair work, mindfulness activities, verbal reattribution, behavioural experiments, and so on). Who is best placed to decide when and in what order these therapeutic activities should be carried out? And how could I reconcile the fact that descriptions of *how* the therapies work varied so widely between approaches? None of the answers I found to these questions were particularly satisfactory.

In 2013, I began working as a psychological therapist for a clinical trial of a novel cognitive behavioural therapy for people diagnosed with bipolar disorder. The study was led by Warren and his colleague, Sara Tai. The approach being evaluated integrated conventional CBT ideas with elements drawn from PCT. I remembered the paper Warren had written and read it again, along with other papers about PCT, including the work of PCT's originator, Bill Powers. Not long afterwards, I made contact with Tim Carey, who was the first person to develop a psychotherapy based on PCT principles, called the Method of Levels (MOL) (Carey, 2006). In addition to reading everything I could find on the subject of PCT and MOL, I started attending MOL training and clinical supervision sessions delivered by Tim, Warren, and Sara. Soon after, I made contact with Vyv Huddy, and we started to deliver our own training on MOL.

What really appealed to me about MOL as a therapy was the extent to which it was firmly grounded in the fundamental principles of PCT. It quickly became apparent to me, however, that the implications of PCT went far beyond informing what an effective psychotherapy should look like (although that is clearly an important issue in itself). If we understand health to be a state in which people can control important aspects of their experience satisfactorily, for example, then PCT can help us think about how we design mental health services to make them as helpful as possible; by making them resources that people can use in order to maintain control over those things that they consider to be important. More widely, we can use PCT to consider issues such as the kinds of communities we want to live in, and what sort of society we want to create. The potential applications of PCT seemed limitless.

In 2016, I was awarded a Clinical Doctoral Research Fellowship by the National Institute for Health and Care Research. This enabled me to complete a PhD in Clinical Psychology that explored the use of MOL for people using Early Intervention in Psychosis services. Since completing my PhD, my research has continued to focus on how PCT can be applied to improve outcomes and experiences for people using mental health services.

Writing this book has been a great opportunity to think in depth about how PCT might contribute to improving secondary mental healthcare. I was delighted that Stuart Eaton and Jasmine Waldorf were able to join the writing team so that the book is informed by their experiences of using mental health services. Ultimately, I hope this book contributes to the development of a new perspective for understanding mental health difficulties – which all of us can encounter at times in our lives – in order to create mental health services that are more capable of helping people live the lives that they want to.

Vyv Huddy

In 2012 I was working hard to set up a pilot mental health service in two south London prisons. The service remit was to enable people experiencing psychosis to be identified as early as possible and supported with psychological interventions. It had been a big change for me, and I struggled with implementing traditional CBT in this noisy, chaotic, and charged atmosphere. I changed tack and tried an approach to CBT for psychosis that was pioneered in veterans' hospitals in the United States. This way of working encouraged a light touch approach and seemed to help the talking therapy sessions to get started. The approach suggested a central role for awareness in bringing about change, specifically what was termed self-reflectivity – which referred to the most basic ability to think about one's own thoughts and feelings. This was conceived to occur in a hierarchy with some self-reflectivity considered to be more complex than others. The task of therapy was to support people to develop greater levels of this 'good stuff'. The trouble was, I didn't have long enough with most of the people I met to help them do this, even if it was possible, and I was becoming increasingly sceptical that it was. The key thing that resonated with me was that awareness was important somehow. But I didn't know at that point why awareness is so critical to how people move from states of distress and anguish, to resolving them.

Whilst I was doing work in the prison I was also working as an academic. One topic that interested me at the time was how people think their way through emotional problems and to what extent imagination played a role in this. In the autumn of 2012, I attended a seminar on a related topic, and I had the good fortune to hear a talk by Warren Mansell about Perceptual Control Theory (PCT). I was intrigued by the talk and sought out a conversation with Warren afterwards. This turned out later to be a pivotal moment for the last ten years of my professional life. In the conversation, I commented that many therapies encourage people to adopt some sort of language – this bothered me, I said to Warren, because it seemed we therapists risk putting words into people's mouths rather than help them voice what's important to them in their own words. I added that my recent work on self-reflectivity had allowed me to move on from this, but I was stuck. Warren commented that I should check out Method of Levels – I liked what he had to say about it. Awareness was central to MOL, but this was based on a more parsimonious, coherent, and clinically intuitive theory.

From there on, Warren and I began corresponding regularly and we decided to work on a writing project together, focused on understanding imagination from a PCT perspective. At the same time, I started reading more about MOL and attended a workshop run by Tim Carey. I was again extremely impressed with what Tim had to say. I felt he was expressing things that had always frustrated me about the way mental health services were designed. Crucially, he also had solutions that seemed to be easy enough to implement – given the courage.

This experience gave me the confidence to start using MOL in my practice at the prison. It took me a while to drop some of the goals I'd grown used to; like endlessly summarising or offering my interpretations of what people were saying and what it might mean to them. But through taking these things away, I found that people seemed to have much more space to talk about their perspective on their hardships. Further, it seemed by inviting them to notice shifts in their awareness they could get themselves to useful new perspectives. The feedback from them was so encouraging that I committed to the approach. I took a pause from clinical work for a couple of years and then started working in an acute inpatient mental health setting, using MOL. I then began delivering workshops with Rob Griffiths, and eventually supporting an evaluation of MOL in the inpatient mental health setting.

A key aspect of my current role is focused on training mental health practitioners to work in a range of settings – most of my teaching focuses on secondary care settings. There are many aspects to working in this context – supporting individuals and families, consultation with teams – and yet existing books on applications of PCT to mental health services have primarily focused on individual therapy, with some attention to service design. I was thrilled to be invited to contribute to this book because it allows an opportunity to fully lay out the implications of PCT for the design of services and interventions. We can showcase what can be achieved if this perspective were to be more widely adopted. Crucially, we will explore this from the perspective of staff and patients by working alongside Jasmine Waldorf and Stuart Eaton.

There is another story relevant to this book that links back to South London Prisons. Around the time I met Warren I was asked to do a talk on National Prison Radio – which broadcasts just to prisons in the UK – about mental health. I thought my voice wouldn't necessarily cut it with the prison population, as a clinician and, possibly, figure of authority. I pondered on this and decided to put out a message on my NHS trust service user involvement message board to seek someone who'd received care from mental health services who was willing to talk about their experiences. One of the people to get in touch was Jasmine. I was impressed, informed, and moved by what she had to say in the interview. The person asking the questions was someone detained in the prison – it seemed to me that this enabled the conversation to happen with only the essential assumptions, based on considered curiosity and fostering a free-flowing dialogue. Jasmine and I went on to work together delivering training for clinical psychologists and it's been an enriching relationship. As we began working on this book, I suggested that we would really benefit from Jasmine's perspective and am delighted she was able to join us.

Stuart Eaton

I was diagnosed with bipolar disorder 28 years ago. At first, the diagnosis helped me to make some sense of experiences that had coloured my life. But, as time passed, I began to have more questions about the nature of my experiences and how they are managed in the mental healthcare system.

After a difficult episode, I was signposted to one of the fledgeling early intervention in psychosis teams, and I stayed under the care of this team for three years. During this time, I volunteered with the early intervention team and, from the experience I gained, was able to secure a role as a Support Time Recovery Worker. Following a number of years in this role, I started mental health nurse training and, after qualifying, I went on to work as an inpatient nurse, first on an acute mental health ward and then a rehabilitation ward. I then worked as a care coordinator for a community mental health team and an inner-city early intervention team.

The sense of a lack of control is one that pervades the experience of being a service user. There is the obvious lack of control (although often fleetingly) of one's own experiences. This is coupled, however, with the control that is wrested from the service user. There is a constant threat to your liberty based on a body of knowledge that is only understood by 'professionals'.

I began to think about the notion of control and mental health and was drawn to Perceptual Control Theory (PCT) and the work of Bill Powers and Tim Carey. I was interested in the concept of humans adjusting their behaviour to maintain control over their perceptions. In particular, I became aware of the Method of Levels (MOL), a psychotherapy based on PCT. I met with Tim to record a MOL video that has been used to train therapists in the approach.

In my view, the concept of control is never more important than in a healthcare setting, and I sincerely hope that this book poses some interesting questions to help develop tomorrow's secondary mental healthcare services.

Jasmine Waldorf

Diagnosed with bipolar disorder aged 17, at a time when my peers had little to no understanding of mental ill health or psychosis, it wasn't long before advocacy became my focus. I met Vyv Huddy in 2010 through the South London and Maudsley NHS Foundation Trust (SLaM) Involvement Register and we worked together with National Prison Radio, going into HMP Brixton to create a piece on recovery from psychosis, experiences of hearing voices, and avenues for seeking help. This project was the beginning of an 11-year journey of collaboration for Vyv and me in the field of mental health advocacy. Over this time, along with another Involvement Register member, I trained 50 Child and Adolescent Mental Health Service staff and school nurses in a service user-led model of best practice, spoke at the National Health Service (NHS) acute adult inpatient convention, and was invited by Vyv as a guest lecturer to share my experiences of early intervention services and first-episode psychosis, where I addressed first year clinical psychology students at University College London on effective practices and methods of self-reflection.

The function of art in disseminating personal narratives and fostering holistic benefits is hugely inspiring to me. Following a period of voluntary work answering the helpline at 'Moodswings' mental health charity, I founded my own mental health and art not-for-profit, 'Wednesday's Child'. This organisation delivered free or donations-based community workshops. We created a supportive, safe space for those struggling with mental health problems to come together and share positive coping strategies, whilst engaging in creative activities led by emerging artists. In 2018, Wednesday's Child was invited to talk at a seminar in Leeds for NIPS (Nourishing Inspiring, Playful and Supportive), a non-profit organisation that creates events for adults and children, where we championed the holistic benefits to mental wellbeing reaped when carers and children collaborate creatively with one another. Alongside running Wednesday's Child, I worked with children and families at the Whitworth Art Gallery and taught both art and relationships and sex education in pupil referral units and emotional behavioural difficulty centres in Greater Manchester, engaging with vulnerable young people with complex mental health and challenging behavioural needs. I am now a practising visual artist and art facilitator, currently working at the Arts Network UK charity, delivering practical art workshops for adults with severe mental illness.

In 2017 I was introduced to Method of Levels and invited by Vyv and Tim Carey to contribute to Tim's book *Patient-Perspective Care: A New System for Health Systems and Services* (Carey, 2018). I was struck by its radically empowering methodology and felt that, finally, this was a move in the right direction for routine NHS mental healthcare. A therapy predicated on the individual needs and goals of each service user is something I had long campaigned to see, and here Tim and his peers were outlining a practical framework for exactly that. When Vyv shared writing on Perceptual Control Theory (PCT) with me, and I began to unpack the potential it had when applied to mental health services, I was immensely inspired. PCT creates a lens through which to reframe the practice of support services through its unrelenting acknowledgement that each and every patient has differing goals that, when realised, will create a personal sense of relief from mental distress. Its implementation as the backbone of care would create a dynamic re-evaluation of the most effective means for individual healing. I am hugely grateful to have been invited to contribute to this book with my experiences of using mental health services. I owe my life to the National Health Service (NHS), and it is with compassion to practitioners of mental healthcare that I lay out my view that change is needed if services are to evolve in tune with the needs of patients. Applying the principles of PCT to our understanding of issues like ward dynamics allows us to adapt to meet the needs of patients by providing a greater level of thought into how we ascertain what the goals of those individuals' might be. It has been a labour of love to contribute to this text. My co-authors' drive to include the experiences of Stuart and me is testimony to their service user-led approach.

Warren Mansell

At the turn of the millennium, when I began my training as a clinical psychologist, my first placement was at the Bethlem Royal Hospital in London. The hospital was founded in 1247 and became the origin of the word 'bedlam', meaning 'a place or situation of chaos and confusion' – complete loss of control – the antithesis of what we, as humans, typically strive for in life. When I worked on psychiatric wards, the situation was never this extreme, but it was not ideal. The psychiatrists were very approachable and knowledgeable, but they clearly held the authority, and their assumptions regarding diagnosis and medical treatment were rarely open for change. The multidisciplinary team valued the contributions of psychologists, but we all tended to assume this would work by 'allocating' a psychologist to a patient for regular sessions. Yet the more I worked in this context, the more I realised that we, as professionals, had set up and maintained a system that limits the opportunities that patients could have to get the kinds of psychological support they want and need.

I had discovered Perceptual Control Theory (PCT) a few years before I started training, but I hadn't realised its transformative potential. Then, in 2005, when Tim Carey invited me to shadow him delivering Method of Levels (MOL) in primary care, its implications became much clearer. People with lived experience of mental health problems need to tell us what it is they want and need. As scientific practitioners, we use the concepts of science to help build and maintain mental health services, but the science we choose needs to be the basics – not 'getting in the way' of any reasonable patient preference – it needs to be parsimonious, agile, and efficient. But maybe most importantly, it needs to be grounded in a fundamental observation of nature. Other theories choose learned behaviour, thinking processes, or emotional regulation as their grounding phenomenon. PCT uses control.

I began to discover that if I consistently ask myself the questions, "What am I trying to control right now? What might other people be trying to control?", then the answers revealed new opportunities to provide support, whereas asking only about learned behaviour, thinking, or emotional states often seemed to lead to a cul-de-sac, and a responsibility for the psychologist to offer the solution. In contrast, asking authentically curious and present moment questions, as we do in MOL, seemed to open up people to explore what bothered them right now, and forge their own solutions.

At least a decade ago, Sara Tai, myself, and other colleagues had started writing a therapy manual for people with a diagnosis of bipolar disorder. It was based partly on PCT, but had focused on understanding and managing mood swings, and it tended to stick to the structure of traditional cognitive behavioural therapy. Our model of mood swings turned out to receive robust empirical support, but the therapy itself, on the other hand, didn't show clear superiority to the other forms of support and treatment that people with a bipolar disorder had received. Rather than stick to the therapy, or even adapt it, we decided to embrace what people in recovery were telling us – provide the kind of support we need when we need it – and to do this we needed a universal, patient-led approach; we needed MOL as a one-to-one conversation and we needed to return to PCT to reconsider the design of services. Rob Griffiths and Vyv Huddy joined us on this enterprise along with Stuart Eaton and Jasmin Waldorf who provided the essential accounts of their lived experience and their own recommendations. Rob took the lead in writing the book, owing to his long-standing experience of working in secondary mental healthcare and his acute grasp of PCT. This book is our attempt to condense this experience to square the science and lived experience of mental health service design.

References

Carey, T. A. (2006). *The method of levels: How to do psychotherapy without getting in the way*. Living Control Systems Publishing.

Carey, T. A. (2018). Carey, T. A. (2018). *Patient-perspective care: A new paradigm for health systems and services*. Routledge.

Mansell, W. (2005). Mansell, W. (2005). Control theory and psychopathology: An integrative approach. *Psychology and Psychotherapy: Theory, Research and Practice*, *78*(2), 141–178. https://doi.org/10.1348/147608304X21400

Acknowledgements

We would like to acknowledge the valuable contributions made by Dr David Shiers and Pru Waldorf to Chapter 7. We would also like to thank Professor Sara Tai, who was involved in the early stages of planning of this book and contributed many useful ideas that helped to shape its development. Paul Devlin contributed to the vignette discussed in Chapter 5. Finally, we are grateful to Nicholas Young for designing the book's cover image.

Chapter 1

Introducing an Approach to Secondary Mental Healthcare that Is Informed by Perceptual Control Theory Principles

Introduction

In this book, we seek to explore how a theory of human behaviour – Perceptual Control Theory (PCT; Powers, 1973, 2005) – might inform the design of mental health services and the practice of health and social care professionals who work within them. While many people find support from secondary mental healthcare helpful, this is by no means everyone's experience. As we discuss in this chapter, many people report that services are, amongst other problems, inflexible, impersonal, coercive, and insufficiently focused on addressing the priorities of patients. This is particularly concerning, given the huge amount of resources that are expended to deliver these services. We are aware that numerous books, articles, policy documents, and treatment guidelines have been written with the aim of addressing the problems that exist within secondary mental healthcare. Where we believe our approach differs, however, is that we begin with some fundamental assumptions, grounded in PCT, about the nature of living things. This informs our approach to understanding mental health problems and the role that health professionals can play in addressing them. We then consider the implications of these assumptions for creating mental health services that can meet the needs of the people who use them.

We want to make a brief point about the language used in this book. Various terms have been proposed to describe people who are accessing support from mental health services, including patient, service user, client, consumer, and survivor. People will have different reasons for preferring one term over another. Our overall preference would be to use the term 'person'. For the sake of clarity, however, it has been necessary for us to distinguish between people providing and people receiving mental healthcare. We have generally opted to use the term 'patient' because there is evidence that this is the term preferred by people accessing support from mental health services (Simmons et al., 2010) and because of arguments that possible alternative terms are associated with unintentional harms, such as being experienced as discriminating or patronising (Priebe, 2021).

DOI: 10.4324/9781003041344-1

Is a new approach to mental healthcare really needed?

Some readers might question whether a radical overhaul of current approaches to secondary mental healthcare, such as the one described in this book, is actually warranted. Where is the evidence, for example, that mental health services are failing to adequately meet the needs of the people who use them? There would be very little impetus for change if the current situation was working well for everyone involved. To explore whether the call for fundamental change is justified, we will begin this chapter by exploring the experiences of people who have used mental health services and highlight some of the difficulties produced by the current system.

Another reservation readers might have is with our assertion in later chapters that it is possible to simultaneously improve peoples' experiences of mental health services while also using available resources more efficiently. Given that a common response to failing or inadequate services is to call for increased funding and resources, this argument might appear unrealistic. While we strongly agree that mental health services should be adequately funded, we also believe that the approach we are proposing could use existing resources more efficiently.

Over the course of this book, we will critically examine existing conceptualisations of psychological distress, along with other ideas and practices that currently underpin the delivery of mental health services. Some readers might wonder whether a reappraisal of the conceptual foundations of mental health practice is truly necessary. Our assertion, however, is that insufficient attention is currently paid to the theoretical assumptions that inform mental health service design and delivery. There appears to be a greater focus on doing what appears to work, with less attention paid to *how* or *why* particular interventions or approaches to service design might achieve desired outcomes. What is required, from our perspective, are services that are informed by clear theoretical principles regarding the nature of human health, including mental health, and an understanding of the role that mental health services can play in supporting these. The principles that have informed this book have their basis in PCT. We will argue that the application of a small number of principles derived from PCT can be used to create an approach to delivering secondary mental healthcare that supports people to live the lives that they want to. Before describing this theory, however, we will first define what we mean by secondary mental healthcare and explore people's experiences of engaging with these services as they are currently delivered.

Defining secondary mental healthcare

The term 'secondary mental healthcare' encompasses a diverse range of services that aim to improve peoples' mental health and wellbeing. Although not an exhaustive list, community mental health teams, assertive outreach teams, mental health inpatient services, crisis resolution and home treatment teams, and early intervention in psychosis services would usually be included under the umbrella heading of secondary care mental health services. These services are generally multidisciplinary in nature, comprising professionals from a variety of disciplines, including psychiatry, nursing, clinical psychology, occupational therapy, and social work backgrounds. They are considered distinct from primary care services, such as those provided by general practitioners, which are generally the first point of contact for those seeking healthcare. There are some similarities in terms of the diagnoses that tend to be received by people using primary and secondary mental healthcare services (Graca et al., 2013; Hepgul et al., 2016; Keown et al., 2002). People who have received diagnoses of either 'depressive disorder' or 'personality disorder', for example, are prevalent in both primary and secondary services. Those using secondary mental healthcare, however, are more likely to attract diagnoses that have conventionally been categorised under the heading of 'severe mental illnesses', such as schizophrenia and bipolar affective disorder.

The financial costs of secondary mental healthcare

The financial costs of delivering secondary mental healthcare are substantial. Between 2022 and 2023, for example, the National Health Service in England planned to spend a total of £15.56 billion on the provision of mental healthcare (NHS England, 2023). While only a proportion of this budget was allocated to secondary mental healthcare, the costs of delivering these services are still significant. In the case of specialist early intervention in psychosis services alone, for example, spending for the 2022 to 2023 period was predicted to be £234 million (NHS England, 2023). Given the significant costs involved in the delivery of these services, therefore, it is important that those responsible for the planning and provision of secondary mental healthcare ensure that it is delivered in the most effective and efficient manner possible.

Patients' experiences of secondary mental healthcare

Research into the patients' experiences of accessing support from secondary mental healthcare is an important source of evidence when evaluating the quality of these services. While many patients report positive experiences of engaging with mental health services, even a cursory review of the available literature in this area reveals that many people's experiences fail to meet what most would consider to be an acceptable standard. Findings from a recent systematic review of 72 studies conducted in 16 countries on the topic of patients' experiences of inpatient mental health services, for example, raised several concerns (Staniszewska et al., 2019). First, several barriers were identified to forming therapeutic relationships between staff and patients, such as poor access to staff, ineffective communication, bullying, and abuse. Second, patients reported negative experiences of coercive practices, including the use of restraint, seclusion, and sedation. Third, factors such as noise and lack of privacy contributed to a sense that wards were unhealthy and unsafe places. Some participants described wards as places that were purely focused on confinement and compared them to prisons. Fourth, patients wanted to be treated as individuals – in terms of their gender, culture, ethnicity, and religion – but this did not always happen. Rather than being a means of improving people's mental health, inpatient services have also been criticised for being unsafe and chaotic places, which offer little more than 'warehousing' or 'containment' for patients admitted to them (Collins, 2019; Fenton et al., 2014). Additionally, despite recommendations that coercive and restrictive practices, such as physical restraint, are only used as last resort, patients continue to be exposed to these practices on a regular basis (Duxbury et al., 2019). This is despite evidence that such practices are experienced as frightening, traumatic, and dehumanising (Cusack et al., 2018).

Problems with mental health services are not limited to issues relating to inpatient settings, however, as the findings from a recent survey of patients accessing support from community mental health services revealed (Care Quality Commission, 2022). Only 40% of respondents endorsed the view that they had 'definitely' seen services enough for their needs, 45% said that they had not been given sufficient time to discuss their needs, and just 47% said that they had 'definitely' got the help that they needed when in crisis.

Issues around coercion and compulsion are also not exclusive to inpatient settings. Changes to the 1983 Mental Health Act in the United Kingdom, for example, led to the introduction of Community Treatment Orders (CTOs) that can be used to compel patients to remain in contact with mental health practitioners and comply with their treatment recommendations (Molodynski et al., 2010). Patients who do not abide by the conditions of a CTO can be recalled to hospital and detained against their wishes.

Further evidence of challenges encountered by patients comes from a qualitative study into experiences of community mental healthcare amongst people described as having 'complex emotional needs' (Trevillion et al., 2022). The study found that participants described exposure to stigmatising attitudes and practices, such as being judged to be someone who cannot be helped, or as a 'trouble-maker'. Participants also reported that services appeared to be fragmented and there was an overall lack of support available. One female participant described how she ended contact with mental health services because of these difficulties:

> I didn't feel my voice was being heard. I actually broke down contact with them because I thought they were making me worse. I just thought I could live it out by myself.
>
> (Trevillion et al., 2022, p. 6)

Reflection 1.1 Stuart's experiences of secondary care

My impression of secondary mental healthcare is that the current system developed in response to the process of deinstitutionalisation. It often feels like another way to warehouse people who, in the past, would have been detained in asylums. I don't think the system of mental healthcare that we have at the moment is designed to support people in my position – that is, someone with a diagnosis of bipolar disorder who is generally well and has only occasional episodes of poor mental health.

My experience of services is that the level of therapeutic input is minimal. Services seem to be focused on paperwork and box-ticking exercises. Every year, for example, I sit down with health professionals and complete care planning and risk assessment documentation. But what is written in these documents doesn't appear to relate to what I would define as the real problems that I want to focus on. Also, the range of therapeutic support is very narrow. The tight focus on risk assessment and care planning doesn't give me the space to think about the lifestyle changes I want to make to stay well.

When I'm unwell and everything feels chaotic it's sometimes helpful for services to take more control over what is happening. Although it can feel paternalistic, someone taking a structured approach to issues like medication, the regularity of appointments, or the timing of admissions to hospital can feel helpful at the time. But this is only useful in the *very* short term. Once I get past an initial, acute stage of feeling unwell, services need to change their strategy and give as much control back to me as possible. This isn't about services unliterally making a decision to withdraw support – decisions about how much services should pull back, and at what rate they should do this, should be taken in consultation with me, but this rarely happens. Health professionals seem to decide amongst themselves how my support will change, and then I am informed of the outcome of their discussions.

In Reflection 1.1, Stuart gives his perspective on using secondary mental healthcare services. Some of the themes in his account relate to how mental health services can be perceived as inflexible, paternalistic, and focused on priorities that do not reflect the concerns of the patient.

In reflection 1.2, Jasmine explores the impact of receiving a change in diagnosis, and how this resulted in her exclusion from accessing some forms of support that she thought might have been beneficial. This is a good example of how judgements about what kinds of support are suitable for certain people are often made by mental health services and practitioners, rather than by the

Reflection 1.2 Jasmine's experience of secondary care

In 2020, I became very unwell following two bereavements and a medication mix-up which led to me being prescribed incorrect medication by my pharmacy. I met with a health professional on Zoom following an episode of psychosis for which I narrowly avoided hospitalisation. In this one-hour Zoom session, the clinician, whom I had never met before, diagnosed me with borderline personality disorder (BPD). I was left feeling very confused and my family were frustrated and angry. They felt that my psychotic episode had been directly caused by me missing medication (through the pharmacy mix up) and the recent deaths I had experienced.

My mum expressed frustration that I could be diagnosed with a new illness so quickly and seemingly with so little insight into my mental health. When I was diagnosed with bipolar disorder it was a positive experience. It gave me an answer to my distress and enabled me to view myself with compassion; I am not 'broken', 'crazy', or 'troubled'. Rather, I have a treatable illness that shapes my emotional landscape and gives me a different set of limitations and strengths to someone living without bipolar. I can make adjustments to the way I live. For example, ensuring I get a lot of rest and a minimum of ten hours sleep is something I have found that keeps me stable. I learned over time what is important to me, how to navigate life and stay well. I thought maybe the final puzzle piece could be this new diagnosis, and that studying coping mechanisms for sufferers of BPD might help me avoid further psychotic episodes.

I began to look up common symptoms and indicators of BPD. Nothing resonated with me. I felt that the common behavioural and interpersonal experiences of people with BPD differed vastly from my experiences and symptoms. This left me feeling confused, so I decided to seek support through an NHS support group for people with borderline personality disorder, only to be rejected as I didn't fit the criteria for the group because I had no history of self-harm.

To be diagnosed with an illness and then excluded from services designed to treat it is hugely alienating. The entire experience was disempowering and isolating. Diagnoses should only happen following extensive contact and work or a period of significant demonstration of core symptoms, I feel that the clinician who diagnosed me did little to hear the recent traumas I had experienced and the physiological effect of taking the wrong medication, and instead focused on me being so affected by death, leading her to assume that my navigation of interpersonal relationships is a symptom of BPD. Being diagnosed has a huge impact on the way you are treated and perceived by those around you, and this was not considered.

patients who are seeking support. Jasmine raises the point that the process of diagnosis should be carried out carefully and sensitively. We also think there is a question about whether diagnosis should be used as a means of determining the suitability of different kinds of support, even in situations where the process of giving a diagnosis is carried out more carefully. Over the course of this book, we will revisit the issues that patients have identified with current approaches to secondary mental healthcare, both in community and inpatient settings, and consider how the adoption of PCT principles might provide a pathway to addressing many of these problems.

Perceptual Control Theory

Perceptual Control Theory (PCT) is a theory of behaviour that was developed by William T. Powers (Powers et al., 1960a, 1960b; Powers, 1973, 2005). The theory describes how living things, including humans, maintain preferred perceptual states through the process of negative feedback control. Before we describe how PCT might help to address problems in secondary mental healthcare, it is important to explain the model in more depth.

Figure 1.1 shows a single control unit as described by PCT. Everything represented above the grey line is proposed to lie inside the controlling organism. Features below the grey line are present outside of the organism in the environment. If we begin with the *input function*, this converts perceived features of the environment into a *perceptual signal*. The perceptual signal describes the current state of one variable within the environment that is currently being controlled by the organism. A *comparator* function compares the perceptual signal to a *reference signal*, which specifies the desired state of the perceptual signal. An *error signal* is subsequently produced that specifies the amount and direction of difference that exists between the reference and perceptual signals. The error signal is calculated according to the following formula:

$$error = reference - perception$$

The error signal passes to an *output function* that converts the state of the signal inside the organism into an *output quantity* that affects the state of the variable under control. The signal ultimately passes outside of the organism and is altered via a *feedback function* within the environment. The change in the controlled variable in the environment alters the *input quantity*, which is detected by the input function, and so the process continues. Environmental *disturbances* will also have an impact on the input quantity.

Before moving on, it is worth highlighting a couple of important points about the PCT model. Even though we have just described this process in a stepwise, sequential manner, in reality, this is not how living control systems work. The sequence of events illustrated in Figure 1.1 are, in fact, all occurring

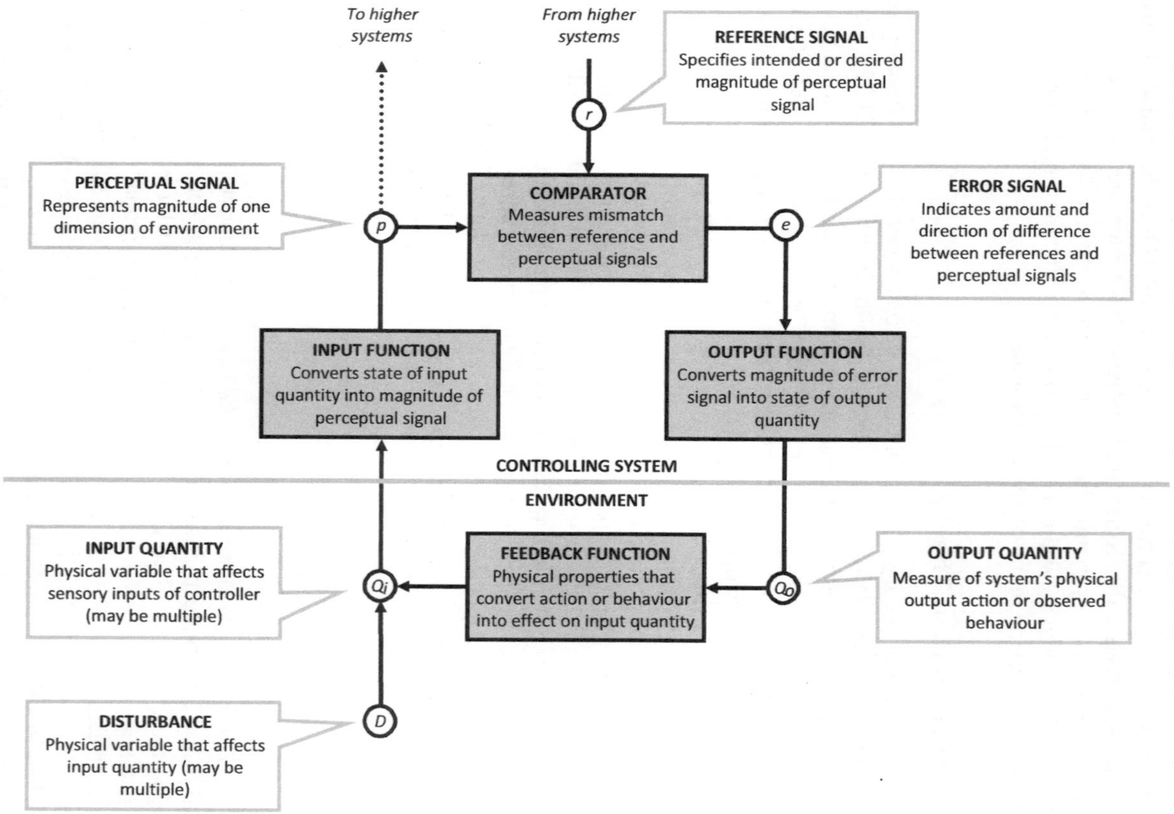

Figure 1.1 A negative feedback control unit as proposed by PCT Diagram adapted from original versions by Dag Forrsell and William T. Powers.

simultaneously as part of the ongoing, uninterrupted process of control. The process of comparing reference and perceptual signals, for example, is happening at exactly the same time as the input quantity is passing to the input function. Another feature to highlight with the PCT model, which distinguishes it from alternative models of human behaviour, is that it proposes that organisms are controlling their perceptual inputs, not their behavioural outputs. Put more simply, we are controlling what we perceive, not what we do.

To make the process of control described here sound less abstract, we will describe this process in relation to a practical example. Imagine you have the goal of paddling a canoe from one side of a lake to another. In this situation, you compare your current perception of your location on the lake (perceptual signal) with your desired location (reference signal). Assuming you have not yet arrived at your desired location, this produces an error signal that specifies how far away you are from your goal. The output function converts the error signal into an output quantity that is sent to your muscles so that you continue to keep paddling towards your goal. The canoe and paddle represent part of the feedback function that enable your actions to impact on your current perception of your location on the lake. All the while, you are counteracting environmental disturbances, such as a strong headwind or choppy waters, that also have an effect on the variable that is being controlled: your current location. This process continues until you reach your desired destination, or until you shift to pursue an alternative goal.

At this point, we need to highlight another important feature of the PCT model. Figure 1.1 is a diagram of a single control unit. Powers proposed that complex organisms, such as humans, contain a multitude of control units that are organised in a parallel and hierarchical arrangement. The control unit shown in Figure 1.1 represents the lowest level within the hierarchy, where the output passes to the environment. In the diagram, you can see that, in addition to passing to the comparator, the perceptual signal is also being directed to higher-level systems. This signal represents the input quantity for the input functions of higher-level control units. Similarly, the diagram shows that the reference signal has reached the comparator from higher-level systems. The model proposes that reference signals are specified by the output quantity of higher-level systems.

According to PCT, control systems lower in the hierarchy are responsible for the control of simpler perceptions. At the lowest level, for example, are control systems capable of controlling the *intensity* of perceptions (e.g., brightness of light or volume of sound). As we progress higher in the hierarchy, we reach systems that can control more complex perceptions, such as *sensations* (e.g., the taste of food), *configurations* (e.g., the shape of an object), and *transitions* (e.g., the speed that an object moves). At the highest levels, are perceptions of *principles* (e.g., always tell the truth) and *system concepts* that comprise multiple principle-level perceptions (e.g., a sense of identity). Irrespective of the perception's level of complexity, however, it is subject to the same process of negative feedback control.

Evidence for the PCT model of human behaviour

The empirical basis for PCT has been described in detail elsewhere (Mansell, 2020, 2021; Parker et al., 2020). Before summarising the evidence, it is vital to remember that the principles of PCT provide a deep and wide-ranging critique of the methods used in the behavioural sciences and in mental health research. Mansell and Huddy (2018) describe a series of criticisms, including the reliance on verbally specified theories, attributing causality from bivariate relationships, arbitrary separation of behaviour, and extrapolation from group averages to individuals. They provide a set of recommendations for improving research methods based on the principles underpinning PCT. But having set these standards, they should be applied to PCT research going forward – 'if you live by the sword, you die by the sword'. However, for various academic and practical reasons, this has not always been the case.

The evidence for the main tenet of PCT – that 'behaviour is the control of perception' – is consistently replicated using precise methods, in that computational models applying this tenet to a variety of contexts have shown a high level of fit with observed data. A proportion of these studies have utilised more than one level of control, thereby also supporting the proposal in PCT that control systems are organised hierarchically within layers. The contexts of these studies, however, are typically within the domain of tracking of visual targets or intercepting a moving object. The same methodology has been attempted within the social domain, for example in the setting of work schedules (Vancouver & Scherbaum, 2008) and in the protection of self-concept (Robertson et al., 1999), but these paradigms lack the same rigour as their counterparts within object tracking performance.

Empirical testing of the remaining features of PCT is even more challenging, especially within a clinical or social context, because these features – such as loss of control, conflict, and reorganisation – emerge in real life from complex, multi-layered systems of interacting individuals. There is a realm of convergent, indirect evidence that the lived experience of psychological distress is the loss of control (e.g., Griffiths, Mansell, Edge, Carey et al., 2019) and that goal conflict is related to distress (Kelly et al., 2015). There are also computer models of the impact of conflict (Carey, 2008; McClelland, 2014) and of the process of reorganisation (Marken & Powers, 1989; Powers, 2008). To date, however, no research designs have been formulated to test models of these processes against dynamic, interpersonal contexts. One promising line of research compares the topography of data produced by a reorganisation algorithm that simulates a population of individuals with the outcome data of large populations of users of mental health services (Huddy, 2023). The model shows a similar pattern of early progress made by some people, and the variety of sudden gains and setbacks that are found during therapy. This represents the first attempt to investigate psychotherapy change processes using a functional – elsewhere termed a 'computational' or 'generative' – model. A recent systematic review of the literature found no earlier studies in this area (Carey et al., 2020).

In addition to the empirical work on the tenets of PCT, researchers have elicited accounts of the lived experience of mental health problems and interpreted them using PCT (e.g., Griffiths, Mansell, Edge, & Tai, 2019c), they have elicited accounts of PCT-informed interventions (e.g., Churchman et al., 2019; Griffiths, Mansell, Edge, Carey, et al., 2019; Jenkins et al., 2020), and carried out qualitative analyses of recordings to explore the mechanisms of change specified by PCT (e.g., Cannon et al., 2020; Grzegrzolka & Mansell, 2019). Further studies have analysed quantitative data regarding outcomes (e.g., Carey et al., 2009, 2013) and processes (Churchman et al., 2021; Gaffney et al., 2014). One promising direction in this regard also relates to reorganisation. Researchers have developed a scale known as the Reorganisation of Conflict Scale (Higginson, 2007) that aims to assess people's tendency to allow conflicted goals and background thoughts into awareness, and there are indications that this capacity improves after receiving Method of Levels therapy (Churchman et al., 2021; Griffiths, Mansell, Carey, et al., 2019).

In sum, the fundamental tenet of PCT – that behaviour is the control of perception, which forms the bedrock of this book – is empirically robust but limited in scope. The remaining tenets are also supported through computational modelling, and a wide range of published indirect and qualitative evidence exists that supports the additional principles of this book – hierarchies, conflict, and reorganisation. There remains a sizeable climb required in terms of methodological rigour and creativity, however, to meet the empirical standards set by Powers himself in order to fully test the complete framework of PCT that we have used to generate many of the recommendations in this book.

Book overview

The aim of this book is to consider how the PCT model proposed by Powers (2005) might inform the design of secondary mental health services and the approach taken by practitioners working within them.

In Chapter 2 we introduce three universal principles derived from PCT – control, conflict, and reorganisation – and outline how they might provide a basis for understanding concepts such as health, mental health, and wellbeing. We also outline how these principles might form a basis for informing clinical practice. Control, it is argued, is a fundamental feature of living things, and problems with health and mental health can be understood as problems of control. Loss of control can occur when people are in conflict, and reorganisation – the basic learning mechanism proposed by PCT – is the process through which people resolve conflicted control systems.

Chapter 3 applies these three principles to the design and delivery of secondary care mental health services. We also introduce the idea that it is the patient's perspective that should be prioritised when planning and delivering mental healthcare. This extends to what support is offered, which problems are prioritised, and how support is delivered. We argue for the need to move away from 'treating' symptoms and disorders, to focusing on problems that have been defined as distressing by the patient themselves. We also discuss how services can be configured to help people resolve conflicts effectively and efficiently, and regain control over those things in their life that they consider to be important.

Chapter 4 introduces an approach to psychotherapy that directly applies PCT principles – the Method of Levels (Carey, 2006). We outline how MOL aims to maximise those elements of therapy that are believed to be effective from a PCT perspective. It is argued that MOL is ideally suited to a secondary mental healthcare context because it can be delivered flexibly and is not constrained by traditional diagnostic boundaries.

Chapter 5 considers how PCT principles might be adopted in settings that are designed to be restrictive, such as mental health inpatient settings. Even in these settings, it is argued, it is possible to implement PCT principles to enable patients to maintain control over aspects of their environment. Adopting such an approach can mitigate against some of the potential harmful effects of restrictive settings.

In Chapter 6, we explore the issue of ethical decision making in secondary mental healthcare and discuss whether adopting a PCT-informed approach might inform and enhance existing ethical frameworks. We also consider how PCT might provide a useful theoretical framework to enable practitioners to resolve ethical dilemmas that they encounter in their practice.

Chapter 7 looks at the issue of how PCT principles can be used to inform the approach taken by mental health services to working with relatives and carers of patients. We consider how PCT might enable us to move beyond existing theoretical frameworks for understanding difficulties that can occur within personal relationships between patients and their relatives. The issue of how to resolve interpersonal and intrapersonal conflicts that can occur in such relationships is also explored.

Finally, in Chapter 8, we look at the unique contribution made by PCT to the field of mental health by considering PCT in relation to other contemporary approaches to conceptualising and addressing mental health problems.

Summary

This chapter has aimed to highlight some of the problems that exist with current approaches to the delivery of secondary mental healthcare. These problems include patients not being able to access support in a timely manner or finding that levels of support are insufficient or inappropriate. There is also evidence that patients find current approaches to mental healthcare coercive and restrictive. We have introduced the PCT model of human behaviour and provided an outline of how, over the course of this book, we will apply this model to consider how mental health services could evolve to more effectively meet the needs of people who use them.

References

Cannon, C., Meredith, J., Speer, S., & Mansell, W. (2020). A conversation analysis of asking about disruptions in method of levels psychotherapy. *Counselling and Psychotherapy Research*, *20*(1), 154–163. https://doi.org/10.1002/capr.12243

Care Quality Commission. (2022). *Community mental health survey 2022*. www.cqc.org.uk/publications/surveys/community-mental-health-survey

Carey, T. A. (2006). *The method of levels: How to do psychotherapy without getting in the way*. Living Control Systems Publishing.

Carey, T. A. (2008). Conflict, as the Achilles heel of perceptual control, offers a unifying approach to the formulation of psychological problems. *Counselling Psychology Review*, *23*(4), 5–16. http://psycnet.apa.org/record/2009-03454-003

Carey, T. A., Carey, M., Mullan, R. J., Spratt, C. G., & Spratt, M. B. (2009). Assessing the statistical and personal significance of the method of levels. *Behavioural and Cognitive Psychotherapy*, *37*(3), 311–324. https://doi.org/10.1017/S1352465809005232

Carey, T. A., Griffiths, R., Dixon, J. E., & Hines, S. (2020). Identifying functional mechanisms in psychotherapy: A scoping systematic review. *Frontiers in Psychiatry*, *11*. https://doi.org/10.3389/fpsyt.2020.00291

Carey, T. A., Tai, S. J., & Stiles, W. B. (2013). Effective and efficient: Using patient-led appointment scheduling in routine mental health practice in remote Australia. *Professional Psychology: Research & Practice*, *44*(6), 405–414. https://doi.org/10.1037/a0035038

Churchman, A., Mansell, W., Al-Nufoury, Y., & Tai, S. (2019). A qualitative analysis of young people's experiences of receiving a novel, client-led, psychological therapy in school. *Counselling and Psychotherapy Research*, *19*(4), 409–418. https://doi.org/10.1002/capr.12259

Churchman, A., Mansell, W., & Tai, S. (2021). A process-focused case series of a school-based intervention aimed at giving young people choice and control over their attendance and their goals in therapy. *British Journal of Guidance & Counselling*, *49*(4), 565–586. https://doi.org/10.1080/03069885.2020.1815650

Collins, B. (2019). *Outcomes for mental health services – What really matters?* (Issue March). www.kingsfund.org.uk/publications/outcomes-mental-health-services

Cusack, P., Cusack, F. P., McAndrew, S., McKeown, M., & Duxbury, J. (2018). An integrative review exploring the physical and psychological harm inherent in using restraint in mental health inpatient settings. *International Journal of Mental Health Nursing*, *27*(3), 1162–1176. https://doi.org/10.1111/inm.12432

Duxbury, J., Baker, J., Downe, S., Jones, F., Greenwood, P., Thygesen, H., McKeown, M., Price, O., Scholes, A., Thomson, G., & Whittington, R. (2019). Minimising the use of physical restraint in acute mental health services: The outcome of a restraint reduction programme ('REsTRAIN YOURSELF'). *International Journal of Nursing Studies*, *95*, 40–48. https://doi.org/10.1016/j.ijnurstu.2019.03.016

Fenton, K., Larkin, M., Boden, Z. V. R., Thompson, J., Hickman, G., & Newton, E. (2014). The experiential impact of hospitalisation in early psychosis: Service-user accounts of inpatient environments. *Health and Place*, *30*, 234–241. https://doi.org/10.1016/j.healthplace.2014.09.013

Gaffney, H., Mansell, W., Edwards, R., & Wright, J. (2014). Manage Your Life Online (MYLO): A pilot trial of a conversational computer-based intervention for problem solving in a student sample. *Behavioural and Cognitive Psychotherapy*, *42*(6), 731–746. https://doi.org/10.1017/S135246581300060X

Graca, J., Klut, C., Trancas, B., Borja-Santos, N., & Cardoso, G. (2013). Characteristics of Frequent Users of an Acute Psychiatric Inpatient Unit: A Five-Year Study in Portugal. *Psychiatric Services*, *64*(2), 192–195. https://doi.org/10.1176/appi
Griffiths, R., Mansell, W., Carey, T. A., Edge, D., Emsley, R., & Tai, S. J. (2019a). Method of levels therapy for first-episode psychosis: The feasibility randomized controlled Next Level trial. *Journal of Clinical Psychology*, *75*(10), 1756–1769. https://doi.org/10.1002/jclp.22820
Griffiths, R., Mansell, W., Edge, D., Carey, T. A., Peel, H., & Tai, S. J. (2019b). 'It was me answering my own questions': Experiences of method of levels therapy amongst people with first-episode psychosis. *International Journal of Mental Health Nursing*, *28*(3), 1–14. https://doi.org/10.1111/inm.12576
Griffiths, R., Mansell, W., Edge, D., & Tai, S. (2019c). Sources of distress in first-episode psychosis: A systematic review and qualitative metasynthesis. *Qualitative Health Research*, *29*(1), 107–123. https://doi.org/10.1177/1049732318790544
Grzegrzolka, J., & Mansell, W. (2019). A test of the feasibility of a visualization method to show the depth and duration of awareness during Method of Levels therapy. *The Cognitive Behaviour Therapist*, *12*, e34. https://doi.org/10.1017/S1754470X19000199
Hepgul, N., King, S., Amarasinghe, M., Breen, G., Grant, N., Grey, N., Hotopf, M., Moran, P., Pariante, C. M., Tylee, A., Wingrove, J., Young, A. H., & Cleare, A. J. (2016). Clinical characteristics of patients assessed within an Improving Access to Psychological Therapies (IAPT) service: Results from a naturalistic cohort study (Predicting Outcome Following Psychological Therapy; PROMPT). *BMC Psychiatry*, *16*(1), 52. https://doi.org/10.1186/s12888-016-0736-6
Higginson, S. (2007). *A qualitative investigation of personal change and recovery and development of the Reorganisation of Conflict Scale*. University of Manchester.
Huddy, V. (2023). Learning curves and psychological change across populations: Implications for reorganisation. In T. Mansell, W. de Hullu, E. Huddy, V. Scholte (Ed.), *The Interdisciplinary Handbook of Perceptual Control Theory Volume 2: Living in the Loop*. Academic Press.
Jenkins, H., Reid, J., Williams, C., Tai, S., & Huddy, V. (2020). Feasibility and patient experiences of method of levels therapy in an acute mental health inpatient setting. *Issues in Mental Health Nursing*, *41*(6), 1–9. https://doi.org/10.1080/01612840.2019.1679928
Kelly, R. E., Mansell, W., & Wood, A. M. (2015). Goal conflict and well-being: A review and hierarchical model of goal conflict, ambivalence, self-discrepancy and self-concordance. *Personality and Individual Differences*, *85*, 212–229. https://doi.org/10.1016/j.paid.2015.05.011
Keown, P., Holloway, F., & Kuipers, E. (2002). The prevalence of personality disorders, psychotic disorders and affective disorders amongst the patients seen by a community mental health team in London. *Social Psychiatry and Psychiatric Epidemiology*, *37*(5), 225–229. https://doi.org/10.1007/s00127-002-0533-z
Mansell, W. (2020). *Chapter 16 – Ten vital elements of perceptual control theory, tracing the pathway from implicit influence to scientific advance* (W. B. T.–T. I. H. of P. C. T. Mansell (Ed.); pp. 585–629). Academic Press. https://doi.org/10.1016/B978-0-12-818948-1.00016-2
Mansell, W. (2021). The perceptual control model of psychopathology. *Current Opinion in Psychology*, *41*, 15–20. https://doi.org/10.1016/j.copsyc.2021.01.008
Mansell, W., & Huddy, V. (2018). The assessment and modeling of perceptual control: A transformation in research methodology to address the replication crisis. *Review of General Psychology*, *22*(3), 305–320. https://doi.org/10.1037/gpr0000147

Marken, R. S., & Powers, W. T. (1989). Random-walk chemotaxis: Trial and error as a control process. *Behavioral Neuroscience*, *103*(6), 1348–1355. https://doi.org/10.1037/0735-7044.103.6.1348

McClelland, K. (2014). Cycles of conflict: A computational modeling alternative to Collins's theory of conflict escalation. *Sociological Theory*, *32*(2), 100–127. https://doi.org/10.1177/0735275114536387

Molodynski, A., Rugkåsa, J., & Burns, T. (2010). Coercion and compulsion in community mental health care. *British Medical Bulletin*, *95*(1), 105–119. https://doi.org/10.1093/bmb/ldq015

NHS England. (2023). *NHS Mental Health Dashboard*. www.england.nhs.uk/publication/nhs-mental-health-dashboard/

Parker, M. G., Willett, A. B. S., Tyson, S. F., Weightman, A. P., & Mansell, W. (2020). A systematic evaluation of the evidence for perceptual control theory in tracking studies. *Neuroscience & Biobehavioral Reviews*, *112*, 616–633. https://doi.org/10.1016/j.neubiorev.2020.02.030

Powers, W. T. (1973). *Behavior: The control of perception*. Aldine.

Powers, W. T. (2005). *Behavior: The control of perception* (2nd ed.). Benchmark Publications.

Powers, W. T. (2008). *Living control systems III: The fact of control*. Benchmark Publications.

Powers, W. T., Clark, R. K., & Farland, R. L. M. (1960a). A general feedback theory of human behavior: Part I. *Perceptual and Motor Skills*, *11*(1), 71–88. https://doi.org/10.2466/pms.1960.11.1.71

Powers, W. T., Clark, R. K., & Farland, R. L. M. (1960b). A general feedback theory of human behavior: Part II. *Perceptual and Motor Skills*, *11*(1), 309–323. https://doi.org/10.2466/pms.1960.11.1.71

Priebe, S. (2021). Patients in mental healthcare should be referred to as patients and not service users. *British Journl of Psychology Bulletin*, *45*(6), 327–328. https://doi.org/10.1192/bjb.2021.40

Robertson, R. J., Goldstein, D. M., Mermel, M., & Musgrave, M. (1999). Testing the self as a control system: Theoretical and methodological issues. *International Journal of Human-Computer Studies*, *50*(6), 571–580. https://doi.org/10.1006/ijhc.1998.0256

Simmons, P., Hawley, C. J., Gale, T. M., & Sivakumaran, T. (2010). Service user, patient, client, user or survivor: Describing recipients of mental health services. *The Psychiatrist*, *34*(1), 20–23. https://doi.org/10.1192/pb.bp.109.025247

Staniszewska, S., Mockford, C., Chadburn, G., Fenton, S. J., Bhui, K., Larkin, M., Newton, E., Crepaz-Keay, D., Griffiths, F., & Weich, S. (2019). Experiences of in-patient mental health services: Systematic review. *British Journal of Psychiatry*, *214*(6), 329–338. https://doi.org/10.1192/bjp.2019.22

Trevillion, K., Stuart, R., Ocloo, J., Broeckelmann, E., Jeffreys, S., Jeynes, T., Allen, D., Russell, J., Billings, J., Crawford, M. J., Dale, O., Haigh, R., Moran, P., McNicholas, S., Nicholls, V., Foye, U., Simpson, A., Lloyd-Evans, B., Johnson, S., & Oram, S. (2022). Service user perspectives of community mental health services for people with complex emotional needs: A co-produced qualitative interview study. *BMC Psychiatry*, *22*(1), 1–18. https://doi.org/10.1186/s12888-021-03605-4

Vancouver, J. B., & Scherbaum, C. A. (2008). Do we self-regulate actions or perceptions? A test of two computational models. *Computational and Mathematical Organization Theory*, *14*(1), 1–22. https://doi.org/10.1007/s10588-008-9021-7

Chapter 2

A Perceptual Control Theory Account of Mental Health, Psychological Distress, and Wellbeing

Introduction

As practitioners and users of secondary mental health services, our experience is that there are no agreed scientific principles upon which they operate. Moreover, when principles are used, they are typically either local (e.g., the values of an NHS Trust), not scientifically grounded (e.g., the NHS principle that patients have choices over their care), or not applicable at multiple levels (e.g., to the care coordinator, the psychological therapist, and the psychiatrist).

Our approach to the design and delivery of secondary mental healthcare is guided by only three principles: control, conflict, and reorganisation. These are the three key principles of Perceptual Control Theory (PCT; Powers, 1973, 2005). These three principles are universal – they apply equally to people who are not reporting mental health problems – simple to apply once they are fully understood, and they have the potential to form a common language between patients, carers, clinical staff, managers, commissioners, and policy makers. The principles inform the scientific basis, the clinical practice, and the ethical context of the service.

Control

We define control in a very specific way. It is the 'control of input'. In everyday terms, we take control to mean the attempt to make your experiences the way that you want them to be. Control is going on when you brush your hair in the morning, when you choose what you want for breakfast, and when you do something to make your partner smile as you leave the house. Control is involved in all of the following: basic needs, desires, fears, wants, ideals, rules, and values. Control is about specifying what you want to see, hear, feel, taste, touch, and sense in any way. To control these experiences, you need to keep behaving in some way, acting on the world around you. But because the world around you is constantly changing, you need to adjust your behaviour all the time to keep getting the results you want.

DOI: 10.4324/9781003041344-2

From this simple definition of control unfolds a realm of opportunities for how to approach mental health services and make them more helpful to the patients they serve. We will summarise the list here and then expand on them in turn:

1 *Control is wellbeing*. When a person has control over what matters to them, they are content; when they can't control what matters to them, they are distressed, unhappy, and discontent.
2 *Services should enable control*. Services need to help people control what matters to them.
3 *Control is often invisible*. What you see another person doing is that person's attempt at control, but you cannot know what that person is controlling without further investigation.

Control is wellbeing

It is almost self-evident that issues of control are at the heart of mental health. In fact, often it is being out of control that brings people into secondary care. A person may have lost control in an acute, immediate sense. The experiences of psychosis, in particular, are often defined by loss of control. Experiences described as 'command hallucinations' or 'persecutory delusions' can disrupt a patient's own ability to effectively maintain control over important aspects of their lives. The inability to control one's own thoughts is very often reported. This includes the confusion of 'thought disorder', the slowed down thinking involved in 'depression', or the racing of thoughts experienced in high mood states described as 'mania'. Patients may also experience loss of control in a long-term sense – consistently not being able to live the life they want. Of course, these 'wants' are deeply personal for everyone. Examples might include not having a meaningful job; not being a good husband or wife; not feeling liked or respected by other people; not feeling connected with the outside world; not having the basic needs of living in safety met.

Then, on the opposite end of the spectrum, some states of mind involve an elevated sense of control, such as the 'grandiose delusions' that can occur during episodes of mania. Of course, people never suggest that having too much control is a problem. It is only a problem when it undermines having control over other aspects of one's life. Someone who has a belief that they possess supernatural powers, which enables them to predict the future, for example, might value this experience but might dislike the impact it has on their close relationships or work prospects. Here, the principle of control helps us to appreciate the challenge of trying to support patients whose 'symptoms' actually involve experiencing more control than usual. Patients are unlikely to be motivated to work on a 'problem' that gives them more control and is associated with a greater sense of wellbeing. The focus of how to help a patient, therefore, has to be shifted away from what professionals might assume would be a problem – like a 'manic high' or a 'grandiose delusion' – and onto what patients themselves say is a problem for them right now.

The focus on what the patient says is the problem right now is at the heart of an approach to healthcare that is informed by PCT principles: the patient perspective approach to health (Carey, 2017). Within the secondary care mental health system, it means that services should provide help with the problems that patients identify. In fact, research reveals a very wide range of self-reported problems experienced as distressing in secondary care patients. For example, a systematic review and metasynthesis (Griffiths et al., 2019) has revealed that people with first episode psychosis could report needing help with the following: distressing memories, bodily sensations, emotions, and thoughts; confusion, uncertainty, and dilemmas; loss of sense of self and identity; physical health problems; reactions to earlier trauma and abuse; difficult relationships with family, friends, and health professions; and stigma. Similarly, a systematic review and metasynthesis of qualitative literature relating to the experiences of people diagnosed with bipolar disorder found that sources of distress were not those typically targeted by mental health interventions. Sources of distress included losing social connections and a sense of purpose and identity, experiences of stigma and prejudice, and uncertainty about the future (Warwick et al., 2019). A typical approach for clinical research is to carve out separate treatments for each of these problems. Yet, an overarching theme across all of these experiences, and across the various studies reviewed, was that these experiences were not how the patients wanted them to be; they were far from their desired states; in other words, they were out of control.

We think that it is time to take stock of the evidence for control being at the heart of well-being and lack of control accounting for distress, alongside the evidence that, whilst patients' problems are extremely diverse on the surface, they match this principle closely. The most practical and efficient way to meet patients' needs, therefore, is to encourage patients to work on the problems that they identify, and for the health service to make sure that the process through which this occurs is valid and effective. This is first achieved by using an approach that is informed by clear scientific principles, which is then refined through ongoing monitoring and adjustment. Again, arguably the most important source of feedback is from patients themselves, from their perspective, as to whether the service is addressing their own, specific needs. In Reflection 2.1, Stuart gives his view on the topic of control and mental health, and how mental health services can support or impede people's controlling.

Services should enable control

If control is so crucial to wellbeing, then it follows that services need to be designed to enable control. This principle needs to be prioritised over an array of competing principles, constraints, and motives that may indirectly, or even directly, undermine patients' control. If a patient wants to talk about their

Reflection 2.1 Stuart's experience of control and mental health services

In my experience, control is the most important aspect in my care. When control is allowed to sit with mental health services, I often find that my sense of wellness is degraded. Control is about making decisions about me, that are important to me, and having full agency in this. Unfortunately, I struggle to think of times when I have had this agency, and often the decisions I'm allowed to take feel largely inconsequential. If my views or decisions go against the thinking of healthcare professionals, I will often have to acquiesce to their view. This then feels unsatisfactory and can lead to one feeling in a state of being somewhat 'out-of-kilter'. It reminds me of a Buddhist concept called 'Duhkha', which means 'out of alignment' and leads to a general feeling of a lack of control and contentment, which can then permeate all aspects of my life.

obsession with cleanliness in a therapy session because it is currently their main problem, for example, this must be the topic of today's session. This stands even if the patient does not have a diagnosis of obsessive-compulsive disorder, and even if their voice hearing is what brought them into hospital. If a patient says that they can only cope with talking about their problems for ten minutes at a time, then this must be the starting point for how long a conversation lasts – regardless of whether the standard therapy session is 50 minutes long. But these are two very simple examples. In later chapters, we explore how patient control can be enabled at all levels in the secondary mental healthcare system.

An immediate concern might be that handing control of service decisions over to mental health patients is irresponsible as they do not have the necessary mental state, qualifications, or knowledge to make these judgements. This first answer to this is that, even if a person is experiencing symptoms of psychosis, for example, it does not follow that they are unable to make choices that are helpful to themselves and others. Most importantly, the patient is in the best position to decide when they are ready and willing to talk about their experiences of psychosis, and this is often (but not always) whilst their symptoms are currently active. The second answer to this concern is that patients clearly do have knowledge of mental health problems, along with experience of services from arguably the most informative perspective – being on the receiving end of professionals' attempts to care for them. The third answer to this concern, is that an organisation should give control to their patients (regardless of whether they have mental health problems or not) only to the degree that doing so does not undermine what other people in the organisation, and other patients, need to control. This is the principle of conflict, which we return to later. In essence, granting control to patients is never a problem in itself, unless it entails significant conflict. In conflict situations, everyone involved needs to reconsider what they are trying to control and move towards a suitable solution.

Control is often invisible

The principle of control has an added value for all those involved in secondary care. This added value comes from the understanding of control as the control of input, not output; control of perception, not behaviour. Unlike the vast majority of theories, guidelines, and common-sense notions in clinical practice, PCT proposes that people do not control the actions we see them carry out. They control for their experience of the results of these actions. What this means in turn is that, to strive for control, people will do what they need to do. They will not necessarily choose, plan, or select a particular action, and very rarely is this action carried out for the benefit of an observer. They just 'do' – until their experiences match how they want them to be.

Because of the principle of control, it is an illusion to think that we can understand what a person is doing just by observing their behaviour. It is rarely that simple. In fact, our research group has conducted a series of four experimental studies that have replicated this principle in the observers of simple visual tracking tasks (Mansell et al., 2019; Willett et al., 2017). The participants in the study were asked to watch a video of two people drawing on a whiteboard with marker pens. One was the experimenter, and the other was a volunteer. Their pens were connected by a rubber band with a knot in the middle. The viewers were then asked to work out what instruction the volunteer was following. The correct answer was that the volunteer was keeping the knot of the rubber band targeted on a dot in the middle of the whiteboard. Yet nearly all of the viewers made a whole array of false guesses from observing the volunteer's movements. Some of the more inaccurate guesses included 'drawing a map of Crete' and 'doing mirror image drawing'.

These studies tell us that even when we have all the information in front of us to try to work out what a person is doing, and why they might be doing it, we can still be way off the mark. This is because patients, like the rest of us, focus most of the time on making their experiences the way they want them to be, and not on how they are achieving this, or how their behaviour might look to other people. Potentially, an observer can come to quite a distorted view of a patient's behaviour if they don't try to understand what the person might be trying to control. The most extreme example of this may be during episodes of mania or psychosis in which patients may be highly focused on achieving certain ambitions or avoiding catastrophic outcomes. Patients often find episodes hard to remember afterwards, yet they will hear other people's recollections of their behaviour from an outsider's perspective. This often focuses on the elements that were not as expected, out of character, or even bizarre or risky. As a consequence, the insider's (patient) and outsider's (e.g., family member or health professional) perspectives may well not match up and this can become a source of distress in itself.

Let's shift to a more detailed clinical example. Imagine that you are a health professional, and you meet a patient in the communal area of an inpatient ward. This patient doesn't make eye contact. Then she moves to the other side of the room. She leaves and strikes up a cigarette. She comes back in and shouts at you to leave. She shouts again, this time seemingly at someone who isn't there. Then she freezes – remaining perfectly still. She looks over to you again and smiles this time and asks if you want a cup of tea. You ask her how she is feeling today. She explains that she's feeling a lot better since you took your coat off. This comment doesn't make sense at the time, but when you get to know her history in more detail weeks later, it does. She had been assaulted as a child by a man with exactly the same coat as yours. All of her behaviour that day – the poor eye contact, avoidance, the need for a cigarette, shouting at you and at an internal voice, the freezing reaction – all of these various actions were to serve one purpose – to try not to re-experience the memory of her assault. Even the most detailed record of her actions that day would not provide this answer. The answer as to what the one experience she was controlling so desperately that day had to come from within the patient herself.

It should be possible to apply this principle to every behaviour you witness, in everyone, patient or otherwise. Yet it becomes particularly relevant, and impactful, when we apply it to the kind of behaviours that we struggle to understand: self-harm, high-risk substance use, violence, apparently bizarre and tangential statements, and attempts at coercion. The principle of control tells us that none of these behaviours are just as they appear; the person doing them is trying to achieve or maintain an experience from doing them. Like the example above, it might be to try to suppress a distressing memory. Equally, however, it could be an array of other experiences. To remove the emotional pain of grief, to prevent others from noticing mistakes, or to feel like a perfectly honest person, for example. The answer will be unique to the individual; their own personal 'controlled variable'. In a systematic study with patients, for example, we found that the majority of auditory hallucinations served a personal goal (controlled variable), such as to feel safe, or to feel connected with others (Varese et al., 2016). As we shall see, the point of a secondary care service is not to identify all of the controlled variables for each patient, like a detective. Rather, the point of the service is to help the patients themselves work out what it is they are trying to control in their lives. But this involves covering a much wider territory than the person is currently focused on – shifting the spotlight of awareness to consider other important desired experiences and how to balance them with one another. This is where conflict comes in.

Conflict

We use a precise definition for conflict. Conflict is occurring when the same variable is being controlled by two or more different goals. These goals may lie in different people, or they may lie within the same person. This variable could be anything of value to a person that he or she can perceive and wants to control. It could be an emotional state, such as anger. It could be a subjective experience, such as the amount of care one experiences from other people. Or it could be something more concrete, such as the amount of money in one's bank account. For conflict to occur, there need to be two or more goals for this variable, and these goals need to be different from one another. If the goals are very similar then these goals tend to cooperate with one another, but to the extent that they are different, they will act against one another, and typically, neither goal will be fulfilled. For example, someone who wants to save money for their security in the future and also to spend money now for their own pleasure, is in conflict. Similarly, a person who wants to experience no anger because they worry that they will lose control, but also wants to experience anger to assert themselves against a dominant partner, is in conflict. A patient who wants to listen to the voices in their head for advice and encouragement, but also wants to push the voices out of their head to stop feeling 'mad', is in conflict too.

Once we understand and adopt the above definition of conflict, it actually begins to answer a number of key questions regarding the nature of mental health problems, and the nature of the kind of help and services that may be supportive when conflict is occurring. We summarise these as follows:

1 *Conflict is the problem.* Thoughts, feelings, and behaviours are only a problem when significant conflict is involved.
2 *Conflict explains loss of control.* There are many ways that loss of control comes about within mental health problems, and the dynamics of conflict can illustrate how they occur, making them more understandable and acceptable.
3 *Expressing problems as conflicts can be beneficial.* By framing a problem as a conflict, there is the opportunity to begin to resolve the problem by working out how the two sides of a conflict can become accommodated with one another.

Conflict is the problem

In simple terms, it is assumed that mental health services exist to help people deal with their problems. However, very often, problems are described in concrete terms, rather than as the complex issues that they often are. The most obvious 'problems' to be treated are the symptoms of what are described as 'mental disorders' – such as hearing voices, unusual beliefs, harmful behaviours, substance use, and mood swings. Yet, consistently, research shows that the so-called symptoms of disorders can be present in people without mental health problems, where they don't necessarily create a problem for the person experiencing them.

For example, auditory hallucinations are experienced by up to 20% of the general population, either as a regular experience, or as a sporadic occurrence (van Os et al., 2009). We conducted a study to try to find out, therefore, what makes hearing voices a problem (Varese et al., 2017). We recruited both clinical voice hearers drawn from mental health services, and non-clinical voice hearers drawn from local religious organisations. They were asked to report the qualities of their auditory hallucinations (e.g., frequency, intensity), as well as the degree to which their voices interfered with their life goals. In other words, whether the voices created any conflicts for them. If hearing the voice made them feel like a bad person when a goal was to be a good person, for example, then this would be coded as a high amount of conflict. Results showed that the degree to which the voices created conflict related very closely to the amount that the voices were experienced as distressing, over and above the other qualities of the voice.

The same principle can be applied to the experiences of trauma. Whilst a history of trauma raises the risks of developing a mental health problem, there are many people who have had traumatic experiences who have either recovered or never developed a mental health problem (Carey et al., 2014). Research on this topic finds that people exposed to childhood adversity are more likely to later experience psychosis (Varese et al., 2012) but the effect size of these findings is much lower than for other health conditions (e.g., smoking and lung cancer). Taking an example of one study with a rigorous methodology by Fisher et al. (2010), around 60% of people who experienced psychosis had not reported any past adverse experiences, which, while less than the 75% in the comparison group, still reflects the majority of the sample. The converse was also true for the control group with 25% of the sample experiencing some adversity but later not experiencing psychosis.

In our experience, it appears to be occasions where the conflict around the trauma is severe that the distress is most acute. One patient, for example, had been sexually abused by an uncle as a teenager and this coincided with the onset of her mood swings. As a teenager, the conflict between wanting justice for herself and not wanting to upset her family was evident. She became acutely suicidal later in life, however, when the opportunity of going to court to testify against her attacker was provided. At this point, she was caught between trying to avoid the threats from her own family, who did not believe the trauma had happened, and trying to get justice and safety for others, at last. Her distress subsided only when the accused pleaded guilty, and she no longer had to try to placate her own family, who had to now admit the veracity of her testimony. Throughout this whole time the trauma had been the same. Yet the stakes for and against seeking justice – the degree of conflict – ebbed and flowed in tandem with the distress.

The same principle of conflict can be applied to any thought, behaviour, impulse, memory, or feeling that people might regard as a 'problem'. None of these are a problem in and of themselves. They are a problem to the degree that they involve conflict between important life goals. To take another example, people with a diagnosis of bipolar disorder very often begin to see their good mood as a problem. It is often identified as a risk for 'relapse' by family members and services. Yet is it even feasible or ethical to try to prevent any 'good moods' because of their risk? Our approach is to help patients carefully define a 'good mood' from their own perspective. This approach allows people to work out what aspects of a 'good mood' do interfere with important goals and which do not. For example, the feeling of 'unbridled excitement' involved in intensive creative work may prevent a patient from noticing the real dangers in a situation and therefore impair their need to stay safe. On the other hand, a 'good mood shared with friends' may meet their need for connectedness with other people, but not make things any less safe for the patient or threaten any other of their cherished goals.

In essence, there is a 'law of relativity' that defines a problem. No experience, or psychiatric symptom, is objectively a problem. This applies as much to the use of a particular diagnostic label, or the use of a particular medication, or psychological treatment. It is neither objectively good nor bad. Rather, for each individual, it has benefits and costs in relation to that person's own goals. People are made up of a multitude of personal goals, and even those goals which we are conscious of will not be held in our awareness all of the time. Consequently, helping people – staff, patients, or family members – explore personal goals to enable them to come to a more sophisticated view of any problem is critical.

Conflict explains loss of control

It is important to be clear that conflict is not simply abstract and subjective. It manifests itself in the real world as loss of control, and the side effects of loss of control can be very clear.

First, the personal experience of loss of control is almost ubiquitous in patients' own reports. This includes, for example, losing control of mood (Dodd et al., 2011), of one's own thoughts (Linney & Peters, 2007), and of one's sense of self (Vanderlinden et al., 1993).

Second, loss of control can be experienced as a state of indecisiveness and confusion, because the individual is stuck between two goals, with neither of them seeming achievable. An aversive state of confusion is one that often characterises the development of a mental health episode (Colbert et al., 2006).

Third, conflict is often manifested as an oscillation between pursuing one goal and pursuing another (Carey, 2008). This can appear as contradictory and inconsistent to both observers, and to the conflicted individual themselves. For example, a patient may spend hours obsessively checking and rechecking the appliances in their house, and then spend the following hour berating themselves for being 'crazy' and 'out of control'. Some patients may have eating difficulties that swing from intensive bingeing to prolonged purging, or mood difficulties that swing from indulging their high moods to clamping down on their moods by self-isolation and self-medication. All of these apparently illogical switches in behaviour are more comprehensible once one appreciates that conflict is a normal, inevitable feature of having many important things to control in one's life. It can be just as important to be given advice through a spiritual connection as it is to not be seen as 'crazy'. It can be just as important to get rid of traumatic memories using cannabis as it is not to feel intensely paranoid because of the effects of cannabis. Conflict is everywhere, and the more inconsistency we notice with our patients, the more material there is to work with, and begin to help them.

This brings us to the fourth manifestation of conflict – invisible conflict. It is harder to work on conflict when it is not apparent. This is often the case, for various reasons. Sometimes only one side of the conflict is evident for a period of time, and so people overlook the other side. For example, a patient who has remained out of hospital for years through a tight adherence to routine and medication regime may seem to have a reasoned approach to their mental health. At the same time, however, they experience anxiety and depression on a daily basis, they haven't worked since their last episode, they rarely see their previous friends, and spend hours in the day ruminating over the life they have lost. For this person, they may have worked to avoid an acute episode of poor mental health as a way to not ruin any more relationships or their ability to work. The other side of this situation, however, is that their regime and self-isolation has also prevented their relationships or their working life from flourishing. For such a patient, it will be important to create a context where they can explore their potential reasons for loosening their regime, as well as their reasons for keeping it going.

In Reflection 2.2, Stuart describes his experience of being in conflict and the effects this has on him.

Expressing problems as conflicts is beneficial

Whilst the kind of chronic, unresolved conflict that we have described above is typically detrimental, the process of making a conflict that already exists open and explicit is typically beneficial. Ignoring conflict does not make it go away; but acknowledging it can. The key step here is to have a way of noticing and talking about conflict in services, with patients, families, and staff. If staff can be at ease with being uncertain or undecided, or they can see how their own problems are the result of conflicts and ongoing dilemmas, it paves the way for patients and their families to do the same. This shifts the focus of intervention from some supposedly objective problem (e.g., the voices, the paranoia, the self-harm) to the ways that this might threaten or obstruct what is cherished,

Reflection 2.2 Stuart's experience of being in conflict

I wanted to talk about two different conflicts that I experience in my life.

The first one relates to my decision about whether I should keep taking psychiatric medication. Medication is a hot topic, and everyone seems to have strong views on this subject. My take is that I don't think mental health services really understand the implications of having to take long-term, heavy-duty medication for mental health problems that are hard to pin down.

I take lithium and several other medications. Because of the toxicity of the medication, I require regular blood tests, health checks, and appointments with a psychiatrist.

This creates a real conflict for me. I think the medication works for me in the short-to-medium term. I am more stable when I take the medication, and my family notices that my mental health seems better. On the other hand, in the long term, I worry about the impact of the medications on my physical health and whether this will affect the length of my life. I am conscious of the evidence regarding the poor long-term physical health of people being treated for mental health problems.

I feel pulled from all sides and it sometimes doesn't feel like it's me making the decisions on this issue. This is an ongoing conflict, which I have not yet fully reconciled, and I often feel the pressure from family and health professionals to continue taking medication when part of me wants to stop.

Another conflict that I experience is about my ongoing contact with mental health services. I currently receive state benefits because of my health problems. Health professionals have helped me to apply for these benefits, and I worry that if I'm not in contact with mental health services, my benefits might be under threat. Part of me wants to stop having contact with mental health services, but I don't feel like I can avoid services because of the impact it might have on my benefits. I think mental health services could be designed better to avoid hampering people's growth in this way. I feel hooked into services in a way that often feels unhelpful.

valuable, and important to everyone. In turn, this can shift the focus onto those important values and principles held by the patient, their family, and the wider system.

Later in the book, we provide examples of how mental health practice can be reframed through acknowledging conflict. Most critically though, the aim is to help patients shift their awareness of a problem to the goals that are in conflict. Most likely, this involves a neurophysiological state in which two desired experiences are 'held in mind'; attention is sustained in this area. There is a range of research, for example, that explores the neuroscience of conflict processing in the context of anxiety (McNaughton & Corr, 2004). Therefore, part of what helps a person to express a problem as a conflict is how problems are described by people around them, but part also may depend on their own capacity, at that moment, to take a 'conflict stance'. This is the person's willingness to experience a problem as a conflict and to explore it. Later in the book we will explain how Method of Levels therapy is designed to help people shift and sustain their awareness in this way. There will be many other approaches, however, that may also facilitate this – psychological (e.g., mindfulness training), social (e.g., creating a playful environment), and physiological (e.g., some medications).

The benefits of expressing conflict may tell us something about what makes a person vulnerable to the effects of conflict on a developing brain – growing up in an environment that does not tolerate uncertainty or allow the expression of the emotions that occur when conflict is experienced. The aim of a PCT approach to secondary care is not to detail the multiple potential 'causes' of mental health problems. Nonetheless, the PCT account appears consistent with the known factors that predispose to mental health problems (e.g., trauma, abuse, overcontrolling parenting, lack of parental warmth, emotional avoidance; McLaughlin & Lambert, 2017).

Reorganisation

The third principle – reorganisation – explains how it is that expressing a problem as a conflict can help to resolve it. In all the examples we have covered, it is never the case that one side of the conflict, one goal, is simply 'wrong'. So, a patient cannot simply be advised and supported to pursue one goal rather than the other. To the contrary, both goals are typically held with conviction, and efforts are made to achieve and maintain both of them. The solution to the conflict will need to be a novel approach that somehow accommodates both goals.

Fortunately, the brain seems to have a way of bringing about novel solutions to problems, in the same way that it learns new skills from scratch – by the trial-and-error learning of reorganisation. Yet, reorganisation does not involve learning or 'reinforcing' any new behaviour. Rather, it is the brain's way of making new connections, new ways of perceiving, and creating shifts in how goals are prioritised and balanced over time. Whilst many other researchers have alluded to this idea of reorganisation (Fisher, 2011; Huether et al., 1999), it can be defined more precisely in the context of control and conflict described by PCT (Marken & Carey, 2015). Indeed, PCT reorganisation has been modelled in simulations (Marken & Powers, 1989; Powers, 2008). These reveal the way that control develops from actions that initially appear random and uncoordinated, and they illustrate how conflict can be resolved in a trial-and-error fashion. These models can even illustrate that perfecting just one goal to the exclusion of others can enhance their sensitivity to any tiny error so much that it becomes unstable, attempting to alter the effects of its own actions before they are even made. It is possible that tendencies that might be described as 'perfectionism', 'mania', and obsessive attention to detail, could evolve in this way when the individual is too afraid to risk dampening down their abilities (i.e., they have a goal of avoiding any sense of failure).

According to PCT, reorganisation follows awareness. Therefore, when awareness is focused on the system that is specifying two goals in conflict, reorganisation can make trial-and-error changes that can begin to resolve it. These changes may be experienced as spontaneous thoughts, feelings, images, or new perspectives on the problem. We have analysed sessions of Method of Levels therapy that reveal a shift from 'talking about the problem', through descriptions of the problem as conflict, to higher level goals that often involve values or ideals for the self (Grzegrzolka & Mansell, 2019; Higginson et al., 2011). The spontaneous changes we might expect from the reorganisation of these goals also occur as patients focus more intensely on what seems to be at the root of their difficulties. Resolution of their problem then appears to follow. We have shown in two studies, for example, that people who report greater awareness of their conflicting goals during an intervention report less distress about their problems afterwards (Gaffney et al., 2014; Kelly et al., 2012).

Reorganisation is enhanced when there is loss of control – chronic, unresolved error within control systems. Typically, therefore, reorganisation occurs when a person feels unsafe or unable to be the person they want to be, or when their basic needs – such as connectedness to others, food, shelter – are not met. Yet if reorganisation is not directed to where it can resolve goal conflict, it will randomly tweak and change other goals in a person's life. Thus, people in chronic conflict can experience the effects of reorganisation on top of whatever effects of conflict they already experience. Whilst there is the chance that the reorganising person may 'stumble' on a helpful solution for a while, in the process of doing so, they may appear (and, in some cases, feel) unstable, chaotic, bizarre, and changeable. There is no coincidence, therefore, that episodes of psychosis, as well as periods of traumatisation, panic, and mania, can have an open-ended, aimless, and chaotic quality to them. The person's brain is doing what it can do to try to regain control. Yet change needs to be focused on changing the systems that will make a beneficial difference, otherwise the effects can be counterproductive. Indeed, this process is exactly what is used to induce a 'psychotic-like' state in animals to test antipsychotic drugs. The animals are put in restricted environments that provide unavoidable shocks and, after a period of time, their behaviour becomes more erratic and enters a different state, thought to be mediated by dopamine-discharge (Kapur et al., 2005). And so, antipsychotic drugs may dampen the process of reorganisation.

Taken together, we can see the paradox of reorganisation. It is an inevitable process that occurs when we are in need – when we cannot control what we need to control. In time, it can take us to a new way of perceiving, prioritising, and managing our lives, such that our needs are met, and we can get back to living the life we want. Yet, it is random, spontaneous, and outside our control. We can direct where it acts, to some degree, but we cannot control what thought or image might pop into our head as a result. If we have experienced the randomness of reorganisation in our lives as children, it might make it easier to deal with later in life. Yet maybe nothing could prepare someone for the onslaught of tangential thinking that can occur during an episode of psychosis, when, arguably, reorganisation is striving to reclaim control against a backdrop of unmet needs and conflict. Therefore, it is very natural for anyone experiencing the effects of psychosis – the patient, their family, and services, to 'batten down the hatches' and try to constrain this unpredictable, potentially risky state of mind. Yet if psychosis is the extreme end of a continuum of reorganisation, and reorganisation is essential to learning, problem-solving, and recovery, then we all need to accept some level of spontaneity and change. We have developed a measure, known as the Reorganisation of Conflict scale, to allow people to report this stance towards their thoughts, feelings, and goals (Higginson, 2007).

Summary

For many people with long experience of the secondary mental healthcare system, the tightrope walk between spontaneous, constructive change, and unpredictable, risky behaviour will be familiar. The principles of control, conflict, and reorganisation can make this journey more understandable, and the common framework can improve communication, coherence, and connectedness within the system. In the following chapters, we provide a systematic approach to secondary care that is guided by these principles, with clinical examples within a service context.

References

Carey, T. A. (2008). Conflict, as the Achilles heel of perceptual control, offers a unifying approach to the formulation of psychological problems. *Counselling Psychology Review*, *23*(4), 5–16. http://psycnet.apa.org/record/2009-03454-003

Carey, T. A. (2017). *Patient-perspective care: A new paradigm for health systems and services* (1st ed.). Routledge.

Carey, T. A., Mansell, W., Tai, S. J., & Turkington, D. (2014). Conflicted control systems: The neural architecture of trauma. *The Lancet Psychiatry*, *1*(4), 316–318. https://doi.org/10.1016/S2215-0366(14)70306-2

Colbert, S. M., Peters, E. R., & Garety, P. A. (2006). Need for closure and anxiety in delusions: a longitudinal investigation in early psychosis. *Behaviour Research and Therapy*, *44*(10), 1385–1396. https://doi.org/10.1016/j.brat.2005.06.007

Dodd, A. L., Mansell, W., Morrison, A. P., & Tai, S. (2011). Extreme appraisals of internal states and bipolar symptoms: the Hypomanic Attitudes and Positive Predictions Inventory. *Psychological Assessment*, *23*(3), 635–645. https://doi.org/10.1037/a0022972

Fisher, H. L., Jones, P. B., Fearon, P., Craig, T. K., Dazzan, P., Morgan, K., Hutchinson, G., Doody, G. A., McGuffin, P., Leff, J., Murray, R. M., & Morgan, C. (2010). The varying impact of type, timing and frequency of exposure to childhood adversity on its association with adult psychotic disorder. *Psychological Medicine*, *40*(12), 1967–1978. https://doi.org/10.1017/S0033291710000231

Fisher, J. (2011). Sensorimotor approaches to trauma treatment. *Advances in Psychiatric Treatment*, *17*(3), 171–177. https://doi.org/10.1192/apt.bp.109.007054

Gaffney, H., Mansell, W., Edwards, R., & Wright, J. (2014). Manage Your Life Online (MYLO): a pilot trial of a conversational computer-based intervention for problem solving in a student sample. *Behavioural and Cognitive Psychotherapy*, *42*(6), 731–746. https://doi.org/10.1017/S135246581300060X

Griffiths, R., Mansell, W., Edge, D., & Tai, S. (2019). Sources of distress in first-episode psychosis: A systematic review and qualitative metasynthesis. *Qualitative Health Research*, *29*(1), 107–123. https://doi.org/10.1177/1049732318790544

Grzegrzolka, J., & Mansell, W. (2019). A test of the feasibility of a visualization method to show the depth and duration of awareness during Method of Levels therapy. *The Cognitive Behaviour Therapist*, *12*, e34. https://doi.org/10.1017/S1754470X19000199

Higginson, S. (2007). *A qualitative investigation of personal change and recovery and development of the Reorganisation of Conflict Scale*. University of Manchester.

Higginson, S., Mansell, W., & Wood, A. M. (2011). An integrative mechanistic account of psychological distress, therapeutic change and recovery: The Perceptual Control Theory approach. *Clinical Psychology Review*, *31*(2), 249–259. https://doi.org/10.1016/j.cpr.2010.01.005

Huether, G., Doering, S., Rüger, U., Rüther, E., & Schüssler, G. (1999). The stress-reaction process and the adaptive modification and reorganization of neuronal networks. *Psychiatry Research*, *87*(1), 83–95. https://doi.org/10.1016/s0165-1781(99)00044-x

Kapur, S., Mizrahi, R., & Li, M. (2005). From dopamine to salience to psychosis – linking biology, pharmacology and phenomenology of psychosis. *Schizophrenia Research*, *79*(1), 59–68. https://doi.org/10.1016/j.schres.2005.01.003

Kelly, R. E., Wood, A. M., Shearman, K., Phillips, S., & Mansell, W. (2012). Encouraging acceptance of ambivalence using the expressive writing paradigm. *Psychology and Psychotherapy*, *85*(2), 220–228. https://doi.org/10.1111/j.2044-8341.2011.02023.x

Linney, Y. M., & Peters, E. R. (2007). The psychological processes underlying symptoms of thought interference in psychosis. *Behaviour Research and Therapy*, *45*(11), 2726–2741. https://doi.org/10.1016/j.brat.2007.07.011

Mansell, W., Curtis, A., & Zink, S. (2019). Observers fail to detect that behavior is the control of perception: A computer demonstration of unintended writing. *Journal of Experimental Psychology: General*, *148*(5), e23–e29. https://doi.org/10.1037/xge0000590

Marken, R. S., & Carey, T. A. (2015). Understanding the Change Process Involved in Solving Psychological Problems: A Model-based Approach to Understanding How Psychotherapy Works. *Clinical Psychology and Psychotherapy*, *22*(6), 580–590. https://doi.org/10.1002/cpp.1919

Marken, R. S., & Powers, W. T. (1989). Random-walk chemotaxis: trial and error as a control process. *Behavioral Neuroscience*, *103*(6), 1348–1355. https://doi.org/10.1037/0735-7044.103.6.1348

McLaughlin, K. A., & Lambert, H. K. (2017). Child trauma exposure and psychopathology: Mechanisms of risk and resilience. *Current Opinion in Psychology*, *14*, 29–34. https://doi.org/10.1016/j.copsyc.2016.10.004

McNaughton, N., & Corr, P. J. (2004). A two-dimensional neuropsychology of defense: fear/anxiety and defensive distance. *Neuroscience and Biobehavioral Reviews*, *28*(3), 285–305. https://doi.org/10.1016/j.neubiorev.2004.03.005

Powers, W. T. (1973). *Behavior: The control of perception*. Aldine.

Powers, W. T. (2005). *Behavior: The control of perception* (2nd ed.). Benchmark Publications.

Powers, W. T. (2008). *Living control systems III: The fact of control*. Benchmark Publications.

Vanderlinden, J., Van Dyck, R., Vandereycken, W., Vertommen, H., & Jan Verkes, R. (1993). The dissociation questionnaire (DIS-Q): Development and characteristics of a new self-report questionnaire. *Clinical Psychology & Psychotherapy*, *1*(1), 21–27. https://doi.org/10.1002/cpp.5640010105

van Os, J., Linscott, R. J., Myin-Germeys, I., Delespaul, P., & Krabbendam, L. (2009). A systematic review and meta-analysis of the psychosis continuum: Evidence for a psychosis proneness–persistence–impairment model of psychotic disorder. *Psychological Medicine*, *39*(2), 179–195. https://doi.org/10.1017/S0033291708003814

Varese, F., Mansell, W., & Tai, S. J. (2017). What is distressing about auditory verbal hallucinations? The contribution of goal interference and goal facilitation. *Psychology and Psychotherapy*, *90*(4), 720–734. https://doi.org/10.1111/papt.12135

Varese, F., Smeets, F., Drukker, M., Lieverse, R., Lataster, T., Viechtbauer, W., Read, J., van Os, J., & Bentall, R. P. (2012). Childhood adversities increase the risk of psychosis: A meta-analysis of patient-control, prospective- and cross-sectional cohort studies. *Schizophrenia Bulletin*, *38*(4), 661–671. https://doi.org/10.1093/schbul/sbs050

Varese, F., Tai, S. J., Pearson, L., & Mansell, W. (2016). Thematic associations between personal goals and clinical and non-clinical voices (auditory verbal hallucinations). *Psychosis*, *8*(1), 12–22. https://doi.org/10.1080/17522439.2015.1040442

Warwick, H., Mansell, W., Porter, C., & Tai, S. (2019). 'What people diagnosed with bipolar disorder experience as distressing': A meta-synthesis of qualitative research. *Journal of Affective Disorders*, *248*(January), 108–130. https://doi.org/10.1016/j.jad.2019.01.024

Willett, A. B. S., Marken, R. S., Parker, M. G., & Mansell, W. (2017). Control blindness: Why people can make incorrect inferences about the intentions of others. *Attention, Perception, and Psychophysics*, *79*(3), 841–849. https://doi.org/10.3758/s13414-016-1268-3

Chapter 3

Using Perceptual Control Theory Principles to Improve Secondary Mental Healthcare

Introduction

In the last chapter, we outlined how concepts such as mental health, psychological distress, and wellbeing can be understood from a Perceptual Control Theory (PCT; Powers, 1973, 2005) perspective. We introduced three principles that are derived from PCT – control, conflict, and reorganisation – to explain how people achieve and maintain a sense of health and wellbeing. We also considered what these principles say about how and why psychological distress can occur, and how people can subsequently resolve distressing problems. Building on these ideas, this chapter considers how the practical application of these PCT principles could be used to create secondary care mental health services that are more effective, efficient, respectful, and humane. These principles, it will be argued, can be applied at multiple levels within systems of mental healthcare. At a societal and governmental level, for example, an understanding of the central role that control plays in the maintenance of human health could be used to inform mental health policy. At an organisational level, PCT provides insights into the design of effective and efficient mental health services that could inform local commissioning practices. At an individual level, PCT principles can guide mental health practitioners' approach to their work.

Mental health is all about control

We introduced the principle of control in the previous chapter. Here, we will argue that addressing problems of control is central to designing and delivering mental health services that are able to meet the needs of people using them. Many healthcare practitioners will already be familiar with the concept of homeostasis, which can be defined as:

> a self-regulating process by which biological systems maintain stability while adjusting to changing external conditions.
>
> (Billman, 2020, p. 2)

DOI: 10.4324/9781003041344-3

The term 'homeostasis' was coined by the American physiologist Walter Cannon (1871–1945), but the origins of the idea that living things self-regulate to maintain healthy states goes back at least as far as the ancient Greeks (Billman, 2020). It is through the process of homeostasis that living things maintain important physiological variables – such as body temperature or blood glucose levels – within acceptable parameters. External disturbances, which would otherwise have the effect of pushing these variables outside of an acceptable range, are counteracted to maintain a stable state. From a PCT perspective, however, homeostasis is a specific example of a wider phenomenon, for which we use the more general term 'control' (Marken, 2021).

Rather than being limited to the control of physiological variables, PCT argues that control is fundamental to all aspects of human health. Carey (2016) has, in fact, argued that control and health are intertwined to such an extent that they are, essentially, identical concepts. There have been longstanding problems in defining concepts such as health and mental health (Galderisi et al., 2015; Huber et al., 2011). PCT argues that an organism can be considered healthy when it is able to control important variables satisfactorily (Carey, 2016). The variables under control might be psychological, physiological, neurochemical, hormonal, or social in nature. The crucial factor is whether these variables can be controlled in line with reference values specifying the desired state of those variables. This is one of PCT's most valuable contributions to the field of healthcare. It provides a new lens through which we can understand concepts that are fundamental to the field, such as mental health. What are commonly described as mental health problems, from this viewpoint, can be understood as problems of control. Following this logic, the ultimate goal of mental health services is to act as a resource that enables people to maintain or regain control over important aspects of their lives (Griffiths & Carey, 2020).

Prioritising the perspectives of people who use mental health services

As we saw in the previous chapter, it is hard to discern what perceptual variables someone is controlling by merely observing their behaviour. Central to a PCT-informed approach, therefore, is the principle that the first-person perspectives of patients should take priority when considering what problems should be addressed and what approach should be taken. Current systems of mental healthcare, however, often appear to prioritise the perspectives of practitioners over the patient's perspective. To illustrate this point, we will highlight two examples.

The Mental State Examination (MSE) is a commonly conducted assessment within mental health services. One description of the MSE defines it as "the observation of a patient's present mental state" (Soltan & Girguis, 2017, p. 1). As part of the MSE, practitioners are encouraged to observe and interpret patients' behaviour in order to make inferences about their internal states.

A patient's physical appearance, dress, facial expressions, and speech patterns, for example, are all deemed to be important indicators of their current frame of mind. In addition to enquiring about a patient's 'subjective' experiences of their mood, practitioners are also encouraged to make an 'objective' assessment of the patient's affect (Soltan & Girguis, 2017). This distinction between 'subjective' and 'objective' assessments of mood appears to reveal that the practitioner's perspective is being prioritised above the patient's own experiences of their mental state. Rather than the practitioner having insights into an 'objective' reality that is denied to the patient, however, the practitioner is only truly aware of their own subjective perceptions of reality. The mental processes and purposes of others are unobservable, which is why it is difficult to make accurate inferences about the intentions of others from observing their behaviour (Willett et al., 2017). The epistemological position of PCT is that while an objective physical reality is assumed to exist, we can only experience that reality through our own perceptions, which are inherently subjective. Implying that practitioners somehow have privileged access to an 'objective' reality is inaccurate and misleading. It also has the potential to create harmful power imbalances between patient and practitioner.

The topic of 'insight' is another concept that is often discussed in relation to mental health. Insight, as the concept is commonly understood, also appears to prioritise the perspective of practitioners over patients. Accurately defining what is meant by the term insight has proved problematic (Marková & Berrios, 1992). One recent description of insight, however, argues that it represents:

> the capability of psychiatric patients to recognise and accept that they are suffering from a mental illness.
>
> (Thirioux et al., 2019, p. 1)

This definition seems broadly consistent with other uses of the term within the mental health literature. Osatuke et al. (2008), for example, argue that:

> Psychiatric patients frequently 'lack insight' into, are 'unaware' of, or deny the presence of their mental illness. Such individuals may deny the presence of specific symptoms, the impact that their disorder has on their lives, and/or the need for treatment.
>
> (Osatuke et al., 2008, p. 1)

It is undoubtedly the case that patients and practitioners can disagree about the most accurate way to define the patient's difficulties. Disagreements might also occur about the actions required for a patient to be able to resolve their difficulties. Insight, as the term is currently understood, however, appears to prioritise the perspective of the practitioner over that of the patient. Such is the disparity between the value placed on practitioner and patient perspectives that, in situations where a patient questions or rejects a practitioner's conceptualisation of their problems as being a 'mental illness', this can itself be seen as pathological. There appears to be a kind of pernicious and circular logic at work here: the patient lacks insight because they are mentally ill; the patient is mentally ill because they lack insight.

Conceptualising insight in this way ignores the fact that the field of mental health is a highly contested area. How we understand and address issues relating to mental health are fiercely debated topics. Arguing that a patient 'lacks insight' if they do not accept the label of mental illness or the concomitant need for treatment ignores the plurality of views that exist on this topic. It also negates the patient's perspective on what problems need to be addressed and how this might be achieved.

One of this book's authors (Robert) once worked with a fellow health professional to support a patient who was accessing support for difficulties related to psychosis and alcohol use. The colleague advised Robert that he needed to 'give the patient insight' into his alcohol problems. From a PCT perspective, such a statement makes little sense. While the reorganisation process can be supported by the process of talking about a problem, potentially helping the patient generate new insights into their problems, insight is not something that can be 'given' to a patient. Such an attitude, again, reveals the tendency to prioritise healthcare professional's perspectives over the perspective of patients.

In order to make healthcare services more useful for the people who use them, Carey (2017) has argued that we require a shift to a PCT-informed model of 'patient-perspective care'. Carey (2017) distinguishes this model from the well-established, if poorly implemented (Hower et al., 2019; Robinson et al., 2008), patient-centred care approach, which has been described as:

> a standard of care that ensures that the patient/client is at the centre of care delivery.
>
> (McCance et al., 2011, p. 1)

Carey (2017) argues that the metaphorical location of the patient relative to the practitioner – be it in the centre, or to the left or right – does not address the problem that patients' preferences about the support they receive are often minimised or ignored; the patient may be at the 'centre' of care delivery yet the features of that care (e.g. location, timing, duration, type of care) often remain decided upon by the practitioners in the service. The patient-perspective approach, on the other hand, requires practitioners to acknowledge that it is the patient's goals that are of paramount importance. We have argued already in this chapter that the function of mental health services is to act as a resource to enable people to maintain or regain control over aspects of their lives that they consider important. From our perspective, it follows that the

Reflection 3.1 Stuart's experience of outpatient appointments

I attend an outpatient appointment with a psychiatrist every three months. There is an expectation that I will travel to where the mental health service is located to attend this appointment, which means I have to travel some distance. The service dictates the time and venue for the appointment.

It sometimes feels like there is a punitive aspect to how these appointments are arranged – I have been told that if I don't attend a couple of appointments, for example, I will be discharged from the service. It almost feels like the service is saying, 'if you don't conform to our way of doing things, then you're out, and you'll have to manage things on your own'.

Working around this system is frustrating, particularly when I have to travel so far for what is often a five-minute appointment. I have asked health professionals about using things like video conferencing technology for these appointments, but this request has been refused. It makes me feel like my time isn't valued and I'm just there to 'receive' care rather than actively engage in the process.

Aside from the process of arranging the outpatient appointment, I often feel like the narrative of the appointment isn't set by me. It seems to be set by the psychiatrist and the kind of things they want to know about, such as medication and risk. I would like more control over the kinds of topics we discuss to make sure we cover things that are important to me.

patient is the person who is best placed to determine what aspects of their lives are important to them, what problems they are encountering, and what goals they are seeking to work towards. In Reflection 3.1, Stuart describes his experiences of engaging with outpatient appointments with secondary care mental health services.

Jasmine describes her experience of working with a care coordinator in Reflection 3.2. In this reflective account, it is clear that the care coordinator's views about what levels and forms of support were appropriate at that time were prioritised above Jasmine's own views on this topic. The result of these decisions had a profound impact on Jasmine's life. In contrast, a PCT-informed approach would require practitioners to prioritise patients' perspectives on what support they require at different times.

Reflection 3.2 Jasmine's experience of care coordination

In 2019, my care coordinator decided that, as I worked once a week, I was 'too well' for her to continue working with me. The implication here is that her caseload was immense, and her other clients had greater needs than I did. This situation is problematic in more ways than one. Firstly, she was inferring that my ability to work overrode my need for practical support with daily living. This failed to acknowledge that the support structures around me, of which her role was a core one, were what allowed me to be well enough to work in the first place. It was not long before I became very unwell again and was assigned a new care coordinator. Alas, I was already so unwell that I was hospitalised and my first meeting with my new care coordinator took place in the mental health triage room of my local Emergency Department.

Services must support individuals to realise goals, without these achievements being equated with being "too well" for support. People who use secondary care mental health services may want and be able to work, but still need support in order to continue to function at that level. Services must not be predicated on the distress experienced alone. Working brought its own new pressures and challenges. Had a care coordinator been involved to support me through these challenges, I may have not had the steep decline in my mental health that led to my hospitalisation and resultant loss of employment.

Focus on distress rather than symptoms or diagnoses

Mental health services have typically focused on delivering interventions that aim to treat diagnosable disorders or reduce the symptoms associated with categories of disorders. This has, arguably, been at the expense of considering other potentially important outcomes (Griffiths, Mansell, Edge, & Tai, 2019; Warwick et al., 2019). The validity, reliability, and utility of psychiatric diagnoses, as described in manuals such as the International Classification of Diseases Eleventh Edition (ICD-11; World Health Organization, 2018) and the Diagnostic and Statistical Manual Fifth Edition (DSM-5; American Psychiatric Association, 2013), have been the subject of debate for several decades. Some have argued that current systems for classifying psychiatric diagnoses are fundamentally flawed and should be abandoned altogether (Allsopp et al., 2019; Timimi, 2014). An alternative approach to the treatment of discrete psychiatric disorders has been for mental health services to endeavour to reduce the symptoms associated with those disorders. This focus on symptom reduction has not been limited to research into psychopharmacological interventions. Research into psychological approaches, such as cognitive behavioural therapy for psychosis, for example, have also used symptom reduction as a primary outcome (Greenwood et al., 2010).

The emphasis on symptoms reduction in programmes of research and in clinical treatment has occurred even though there is evidence that this might not be a priority for many people using mental health services. In a study where people with experience of psychosis were asked to rate items as essential for defining recovery, for example, items such as 'Recovery is the achievement of a personally acceptable quality of life' and 'Recovery is the process of regaining active control over one's life' were rated highly by participants (Law & Morrison, 2014). When participants were asked to rate items that help and hinder recovery from psychosis, participants rated items such as 'Having a good, safe place to live' and 'Having the support of others' more highly than items relating to symptoms of psychosis. Similarly, a recent systematic review of 33 qualitative studies that explored first-person perspectives on experiences of first-episode psychosis found that participants reported a very wide range of sources of distress, including distress connected to personal relationships, contact with mental health services, and societal stigma (Griffiths, Mansell, Edge, & Tai, 2019). This suggests that maintaining a narrow focus on symptom reduction within mental health research will not address the priorities of people using mental health services.

From a PCT perspective, internal conflicts do not occur only within the context of specific psychiatric disorders. Conflict has been described as a transdiagnostic process (Carey, 2008b). In fact, it is probably more accurate to describe conflict as an "adiagnostic" process, since all of us will experience conflict at some point in our life, irrespective of whether we have received a psychiatric diagnosis or not. Deciding whether to have cup of Earl Grey tea or a cappuccino is a conflict. Mulling over whether to stay late at work or go home to join your family for dinner is a conflict. As is being unsure whether to walk or drive to an appointment. Conflicts are an inevitable and ubiquitous feature of life. Most of the time we can resolve conflicts without this causing us any significant difficulties – we choose the Earl Grey tea or the cappuccino and carry on with our day. What can be problematic, however, are conflicts that remain unresolved for a sustained period (Carey, 2008a). The result of ongoing, unresolved conflicts is psychological distress, and this is the problem that we think mental health services should aim to address.

While focusing on symptom reduction might appear to avoid some of the issues that have been identified with the validity and reliability of psychiatric diagnoses, this approach is similarly fraught with problems. Auditory hallucinations, for example, are often considered to be a symptom of a psychotic disorder (Waters & Fernyhough, 2017) as defined in manuals such as the DSM-5 (American Psychiatric Association, 2013). There is now good evidence, however, that many people describe experiences such as hearing things that others do not without experiencing significant distress or requiring support from mental health services (Lawrence et al., 2010; Maijer et al., 2018). From a PCT perspective, experiences such as hearing voices are problematic only in situations where this creates conflict. An example might be someone who wants to listen to a voice that others cannot hear because they find it comforting, but they also do not want to hear the voice because they worry that other people will judge them negatively. In this situation, since the person cannot meet their 'listen to the voice' and 'don't listen to the voice' goals simultaneously, the conflict is likely to be distressing. It is the conflict, however, that is the source of the distress, rather than the symptom in isolation. This is the principle of 'relativity' which we referred to in Chapter 2.

Rather than focusing on treating psychiatric disorders or symptoms, therefore, our suggestion is that one way that mental health services can become more helpful is by supporting people to resolve the conflicts that create psychological distress. The exact nature of the conflicts experienced by people will vary widely, but there are general principles, derived from PCT, that can inform this process.

Enabling people to resolve internal conflicts

PCT argues that psychological distress is often the result of chronic, unresolved internal conflicts that are held outside of awareness. A simplified example of a distressing conflict that someone seeking support from mental health services might experience is presented in Figure 3.1. This illustrates a situation where someone is 'in two minds' about whether to continue taking psychotropic medication. This conflict is occurring over three levels. At the lowest level, the variable being controlled is the patient's concordance with prescribed medication. The person's current perceptual input (I) is compared to a reference value for the state of that perception (C). Where there is a difference between current perceptions and the reference for the state of the variable, the output function (O) produces an output signal that affects the state of the variable, with the aim of reducing error. The level above this represents the conflicted control systems. On one side of the conflict, perhaps the person has a goal to follow the advice of health professionals. They might be concerned that going against professional advice and stopping their medication altogether could result in them experiencing further mental health difficulties in the future. This could have serious consequences for other important goals held by the person, such as avoiding readmission to hospital, or to minimise potential disruptions to their career or personal relationships. On the other hand, they might have concerns about the potential side effects of prescribed medication. A higher-level goal to 'live a healthy life' could be setting the reference value for two incompatible lower-level goals: 'Follow the advice of health professionals' and 'Avoid medication side effects'. Since it is not possible to keep taking medication as it is prescribed whilst simultaneously stopping the medication, the result is a conflict that disrupts effective control in this area of the person's life.

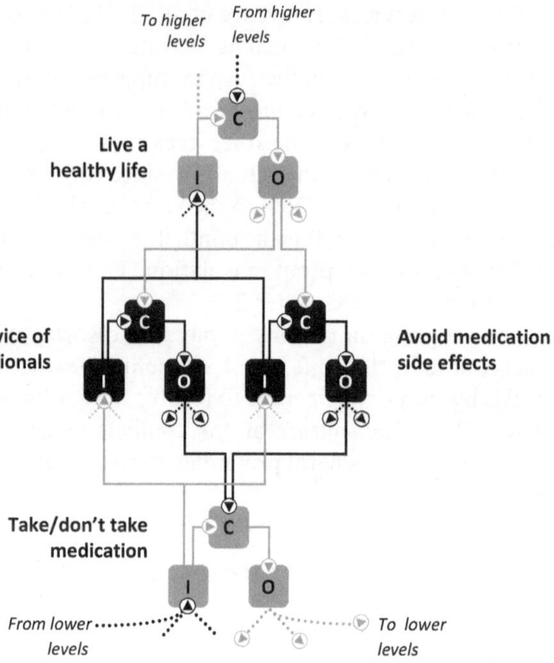

Figure 3.1 Simplified representation of an individual's conflict about taking medication.

This conflict might mean that the person fluctuates between taking the medication regularly, stopping their medication altogether, or taking their medication only occasionally. Impaired control over this aspect of their life has the potential to be disruptive and distressing.

People can resolve conflicts when they are able to sustain their awareness on the source of the conflict for a sufficient length of time to allow the reorganisation process to take place. In the example described above, if the person is given space to discuss the problem in detail – sustaining their awareness on the different facets of the conflict – it is possible that they will be able to resolve the conflict in a way that they find satisfactory. For example, they may be able to explore the mid-level goals for taking medication that serve to live a healthy life at a higher level – to prevent a hospital admission or to reduce risky emotional states, for example. Similarly, they may be helped to explore the mid-level goals for not taking medication that serve to live a healthy life – to remove the side effects of fatigue and to experience more fulfilling emotional states, for example. It would be through a more thorough, detailed, and even-handed exploration of all of these conflicted goals that a person arrives at an understanding at a higher perspective and begins to manage the conflict in a manner that actually achieves and maintains the higher-level goal (of living a healthy life, in this case).

In Chapter 4, we will describe a psychological therapy that is based on PCT, called the Method of Levels (Carey, 2006), that specifically aims to help people shift and sustain their awareness to the systems driving conflict to allow their reorganisation, and thereby enabling people to resolve the key conflicts that are undermining the control of their lives.

Practitioners who are working with patients experiencing conflicts like the one illustrated in Figure 3.1 might be tempted to offer some advice and suggestions about how this problem could be resolved. We have met many practitioners who have strong opinions on this topic – some who are very positive about the benefits of taking medication, and others who are highly opposed. Practitioners are unlikely to be experienced as helpful, however, when they encourage the person to attend to only one side of a conflict such as this, or where opportunities for the person to reflect in depth on their problems are limited. In the situation described above, for example, a community mental health nurse might feel that part of their role is to encourage patients to continue to take their medication as it is prescribed, even in situations where the patient feels some ambivalence about doing so. Given that interventions have been developed with the specific aim of encouraging people using mental health services to adhere to prescribed medications (e.g., García-Pérez et al., 2020), this is not an unlikely scenario. The nurse might meet their goal to 'make sure my patients take their medication as prescribed' by emphasising the benefits of medication or by highlighting potential negative outcomes that might occur should the person discontinue their medication. Since there is a conflict rumbling away at the back of the patient's mind about taking medication, however, an approach that only attends to one side of the conflict is unlikely to be experienced as helpful for very long. Maybe the patient will start to be less open about the issue of medication, or they might decide that it is not helpful to maintain contact with the nurse. Where the patient can have an open conversation about their medication dilemma, one that allows them to sustain their awareness on both sides of the conflict, the more likely it is that they will be able to develop new perspectives on the problem and come to a resolution that they find acceptable.

As mentioned, the Method of Levels is an approach to psychotherapy that specifically aims to help people resolve conflicts (Carey, 2006). We do not think that it makes sense, however, for these kinds of helpful conversations to be limited to interactions occurring within the context of psychotherapy. If unresolved conflicts are what lie behind much of the distress experienced by people using mental health services, then practitioners and services will be experienced as more helpful when the provision of frequent opportunities for people to resolve conflicts becomes routine practice. Practitioners can support the conflict resolution process by adopting an approach that is characterised by genuine curiosity. In practice, this means providing an environment where people feel able to sustain their awareness on both sides of a conflict whilst also feeling able to express themselves freely. In Reflection 3.3, Stuart describes his experience

Reflection 3.3 Stuart's experience of discussions with health professionals

Lots of the conversations I have with health professionals are brief – often under five minutes. It sometimes doesn't feel like there is much investment from the service or professional involved – just a box ticking exercise.

'Are you okay? Yes? Great, see you again in six months'.

Services do seem to react quickly in times of crisis, but this is from a medical perspective (e.g., medication to help me feel calmer). They don't ask what's important to me. When they ask how I feel, these conversations often feel perfunctory. The topics discussed are left at a surface level; they don't go deeper than acknowledging my initial response. There seems to be a lack of curiosity about my underlying experiences. I wonder if this is because of a mismatch between our goals. The member of staff might want to fill in a risk assessment, but I want my life to get better. I don't think there's anything nefarious in this. It's just that the system doesn't currently work to help prioritise the things that patients think are important.

of talking to health professionals where the conversation has been characterised by a lack of curiosity about his underlying experiences. Practitioners using MOL and informed by PCT would spend time trying to understand more about the experiences of the people they are working with and how they can be supported to meet important personal goals.

Our advice is to be cautious about offering advice

Related to the above point, our experience is that many practitioners consider providing information and advice to patients to be an important part of their role. Advice is sometimes given as informal suggestions for activities the patient should engage in to a greater or lesser extent (for example, to get more physical exercise, stop smoking, eat healthily, drink less alcohol, engage in mindfulness, or find a hobby). At other times, this advice might be more formalised and described as 'psychoeducation' (Bäuml et al., 2006). While the advice is probably given with the best of intentions, it actually has the potential to disrupt reorganisation that might be in the process of resolving a conflict and enhancing patient control. Advice offered from the perspective of an observer, however well intentioned, can therefore be unhelpful. One reason for this is that the individual experiencing a problem is the only one who is fully able to appreciate all the facets and nuances of the difficulty they are encountering. Only they have a first-person perspective on all aspects of the conflict. Most of us have at some point had the experience of being given advice by someone and offering a reply along the lines, 'Thanks for the suggestion, but that won't work because …', before going on to explain some other aspect of the problem that would make the solution offered untenable.

Information (but not advice) might be helpful in situations where people are specifically looking for it. If someone does not know the side effects associated with a newly prescribed medication, someone telling them this information could be very helpful. This is a situation where a lack of knowledge about a particular topic, rather than a conflict, is impeding the person's ability to maintain control over something important to them (in this case, their ability to make informed choices about taking medication).

Where someone is experiencing an enduring and problematic conflict, however, giving advice is unlikely to resolve the conflict. If someone is worrying about the effects of their level of alcohol consumption but drinking several glasses of wine in the evening helps them to feel less stressed, advising the person to stop drinking because they are damaging their health is unlikely to be helpful. The person is probably already aware that their levels of drinking are potentially harmful. Presumably, that is why they already have concerns about the issue and want to talk to someone about it. The problem is that they are in a state of conflict, and advice given from the perspective of an observer is unlikely to help them to resolve this. Rather than offering advice, our findings suggest that when practitioners maintain a stance of curiosity about people's difficulties, and provide opportunities for the open expression of problems, people can generate bespoke solutions to their problems without the need for advice (Griffiths, Mansell, Edge, & Tai, 2019).

The change process is unique to individuals

Reorganisation is the process through which people resolve distressing conflicts and regain control over important aspects of their life (Powers, 1973, 2005). An important feature of reorganisation is that it is a random, trial-and-error process. This means that it is not possible to accurately predict when the reorganisation process will result in a conflict being resolved in a way that the individual considers satisfactory. This has several implications for mental health services. First, it means the amount of time someone needs support from services will vary considerably between individuals. Some people might find that they are able to resolve the problems for which they are seeking help relatively quickly, and only a short period of support is required to help them achieve this. For other people, however, finding a satisfactory resolution to their difficulties could take longer, and a greater duration of support is required. Second, because the patient is the only one with a first-person perspective on the conflict, they are generally best placed to make judgements on issues such as when support is required from mental health services, how long the support should last, and the optimum frequency of contact with mental health services. Third, people will need different kinds of support to help them make the changes that they see as being required. Again, the patient is best placed to know what support will be helpful in resolving their conflict.

Currently, mental health services appear to be configured on a 'one-size-fits-all' basis. Recommendations for the optimum number of sessions of psychological therapy within treatment guidelines, for example, do not appear to take the natural variation that exists between people into account. The National Institute for Health and Care Excellence (NICE) in the UK recommend that people with severe depression should receive at least 16 sessions of cognitive behavioural therapy (CBT) (NICE, 2022). Similarly, for people experiencing psychosis, NICE recommends that CBT should be delivered over 16 planned sessions (NICE, 2014). The empirical or theoretical reasons for choosing a specific number of therapy sessions, however, remain unclear, and we are unaware of any research specifically manipulating the number of sessions to quantify the effects on outcomes for different individuals. Indeed, there is some evidence that the relationship between the number of therapy sessions attended and patient outcomes is not at all clear (Stiles et al., 2008). Similarly, UK guidelines for people experiencing a first episode of psychosis recommend that people should be offered access to specialist early intervention services for up to three years (NHS England et al., 2016). This might reflect the average amount of time for the population of people who report psychosis to 'recover', but exactly three years is unlikely to be the appropriate length of support for any one individual in particular.

PCT-informed mental health services would take the natural variation that exists between people into account and enable them to access support in a way that meets their individual needs. Indeed, a system of appointment scheduling has already been developed, which is based on PCT principles, that aims to give people control over the frequency and duration of psychological therapy sessions (Carey et al., 2013). The approach, called 'patient-led scheduling', enables people accessing therapy to choose how often they have a session and the length of time they engage with therapy. The aim is that people can attend sessions for as long as they find it helpful for them to do so. There is evidence that people appreciate the control that this system of appointment booking gives them over the process of therapy (Griffiths, Mansell, Edge, Carey, et al., 2019). There is also some evidence that therapy delivered using this system of appointment scheduling is as effective as conventional approaches to appointment scheduling, but has advantages in terms of efficiency (Carey et al., 2013). We will explore the principles and practicalities of using patient-led scheduling in detail in Chapter 4.

Understanding people as controllers

Descriptions of mental health services can sometimes conjure up an image of a one-way street, a linear pathway travelling from practitioner to patient. Practitioners are said to 'deliver' mental health interventions to patients. Similarly, psychotropic medications are 'administered', and patients are 'treated'. Described in these terms, it sounds as if the patient is the passive recipient of mental health practitioners' expertise and interventions. In our view, however, this view of mental health services risks disregarding patients' goals and undermining their sense of agency.

Understood from a PCT perspective, patient–practitioner exchanges can instead be seen as interactions between controllers. Both patients and practitioners are controlling their perceptions to maintain them in line with reference values for the state of those perceptions. As mentioned previously, the term 'reference value' refers to a person's goals for the state of a particular perception. Put simply, the reference value describes how the person would like things to be. Control is achieved by comparing current perceptions against references for the desired state of those perceptions. Where a discrepancy exists, the person acts to reduce this difference. Since patients are part of the environment that is perceived by practitioners, and practitioners are part of the environment perceived by patients, it is likely that both parties will have references that relate to each other.

Problems are unlikely to arise in situations where the goals of both patients and practitioners are broadly aligned with each other; if both parties agree, for example, that they will meet on a weekly basis to engage in a particular psychological therapy. Where things become problematic is in circumstances where the goals of the practitioner and patient are at odds with each other. An example might be where a practitioner has a goal to discharge a patient from a community mental health team, but the patient wants to continue to receive the support from that service. Here, the more the practitioner works towards their 'discharge the patient' goal, the more this acts as a disturbance to the patient's 'continue to receive support goal'. Similarly, if a practitioner believes that a patient should be admitted to a mental health inpatient unit, but the patient disagrees with this assessment, this is likely to disrupt the controlling of one or both of those concerned, at least until the disagreement is resolved.

One of this book's authors (Robert), worked for several years as a community mental health nurse in an Assertive Outreach Team. As part of this role, he and his colleagues would attempt to visit a particular patient at home on a weekly basis. The mental health workers would knock on the patient's front door several times. Eventually, the patient would open an upstairs window and tell the mental health workers to leave (in the strongest possible terms), before closing the window again. The mental health workers would subsequently return to their team office and diligently record the details of this exchange in the patient's clinical records. This sequence of events was repeated for several months, with very little variation.

One reason for mentioning this anecdote is because PCT provides a framework for understanding the complex and challenging situations, such as this one, that mental health practitioners can often encounter. Understanding people as controllers can help us to make sense of what, on the surface, seems like quite an unusual interaction between the patient and their mental health workers. As we have outlined previously, it is not possible to say with certainty exactly what other people are attempting to control simply by observing their behaviour (Willett et al., 2017). It seems relatively likely, however, that one of the patient's goals in this situation was to not have contact with the mental health team. If that is the case, however, why did the patient not completely ignore the practitioner knocking on their door? Why take the trouble to shout out of the window? It is also not entirely clear what the mental health practitioners were seeking to achieve. What compelled them to knock on the person's door each week only to be sworn at? Why would they continue to engage in this behaviour, even when the patient had explicitly (in both senses that the word is commonly used) stated that they wished them to stop?

Certainly, during team discussions, it became apparent that many members of staff felt uncomfortable engaging in this kind of activity. They described ethical concerns about overriding the patient's freedom to decline mental healthcare. Promoting patient's autonomy and freedom of choice were valued goals held by staff members. At the same time, however, team members acknowledged that they held other important, but contradictory, goals. Examples of these contradictory goals included adhering to guidelines for professional practice, following the policies and procedures of their employer, and avoiding possible censure arising from a perception that they had failed to carry out their duties appropriately. These appear to be relatively common dilemmas experienced by practitioners working in this kind of context (Claassen & Priebe, 2007). In this example, therefore, while there are elements of an interpersonal conflict between practitioners and the patient, there are also indications that at least some of the practitioners were experiencing a degree of intrapersonal conflict relating to their practice.

Figure 3.2 is an illustration of the interpersonal and intrapersonal conflicts that might have been at play in this situation. To be clear, without asking detailed questions of all parties involved, it is not possible to say exactly what goals they were working towards in this situation. With that caveat in mind, what the figure aims to illustrate is a hypothesis regarding how both patient and practitioner are seeking to control the same aspect of the environment. Specifically, how much contact they have with each other. On the patient's side of the figure, there is an indication that they are experiencing some internal conflict. The patient's higher-level goal is to avoid being detained in hospital under mental health legislation. This is setting two incompatible reference values (or goals). One way that the patient is seeking to achieve this goal is to avoid all contact with the practitioner. Perhaps the patient is concerned, however, that the situation might escalate if the practitioner is not able to have any contact with them. Perhaps the practitioner might request that the patient is assessed under mental health legislation with a view to admitting them to hospital. Another of the patient's goals, therefore, might be to have some limited

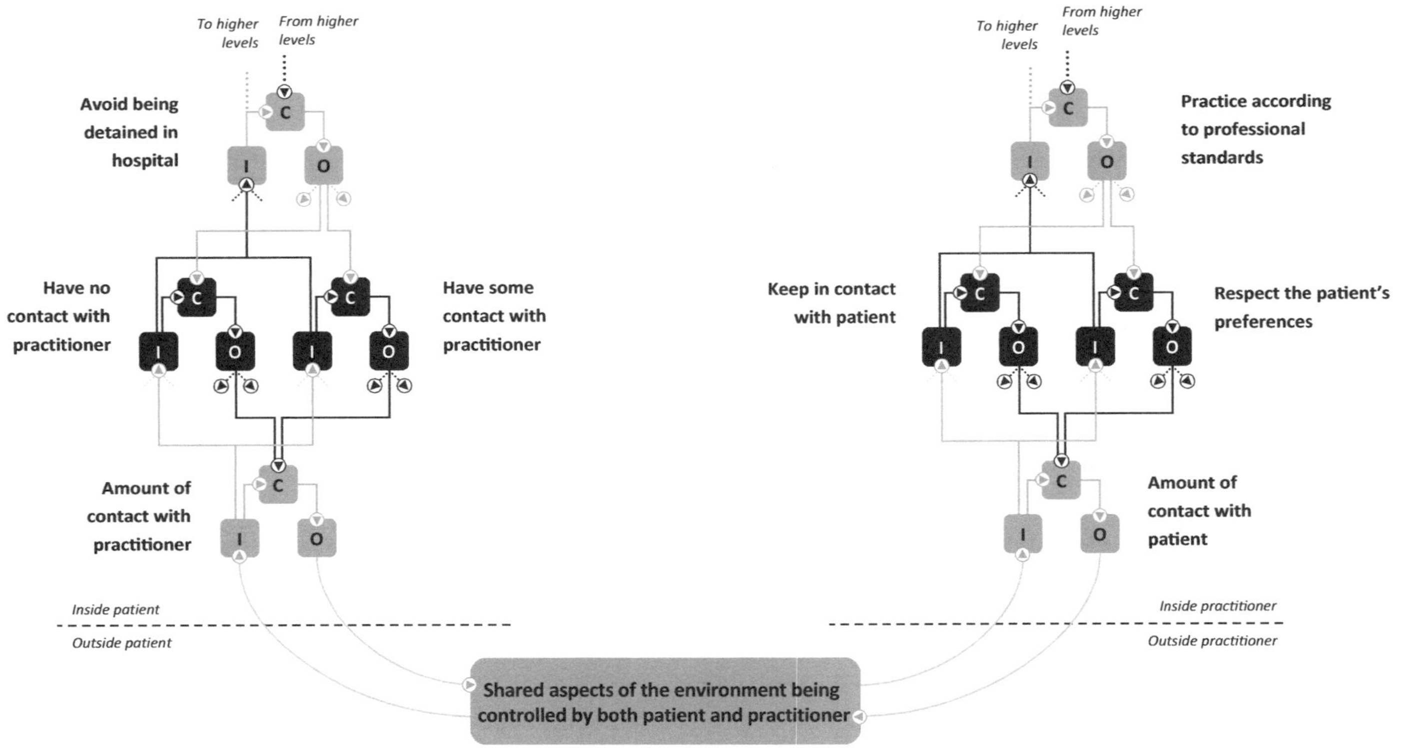

Figure 3.2 Diagram illustrating an interpersonal conflict between patient and practitioner relating to the amount of contact between both parties. The diagram also includes intrapersonal conflicts experienced by both patient and practitioner relating to the control of this variable.

contact with the practitioner, even if this takes the form of shouting at them to go away. This conflict means that the patient is caught between engaging in behaviours such as shouting at the practitioner to leave or ignoring the practitioner completely.

Examining the practitioner's side of the figure, it is the higher-level goal of practising according to professional standards that is setting the incompatible reference values at lower levels. The practitioner is caught between wanting to maintain contact with the patient (perhaps because of the policies of their employer to assertively engage people in this kind of situation), while also wanting to respect the patient's preference for not having any contact with mental health services. This means that they might alternate between meeting these two goals, or the practitioner might prioritise one of the goals but experience some discomfort about doing so.

The consequence of these ongoing interpersonal and intrapersonal conflicts is that neither patient nor practitioner will be able to control the variable in question – the amount of contact they have with each other – in a satisfactory way. For both parties, ongoing internal conflicts will mean that their attempts to meet one goal will act as a disturbance to other goals and vice versa. Additionally, even if one or both individuals concerned were able to successfully resolve their internal conflicts, the variable cannot be controlled in a way that is acceptable to both parties while the patient's and practitioner's goals are substantially misaligned. Restoring effective control over this variable for both patient and practitioner will require the resolution of both the internal conflicts and the interpersonal conflict.

A strength of PCT is that it provides a theoretical framework for conceptualising situations such as this one. PCT could also form the basis for how to approach clinical supervision, enabling practitioners to explore and resolve professional conflicts that might impede their ability to perform their role effectively. Further, an understanding of people as controllers could inform discussions between service providers and patients about their respective goals, allowing them to navigate possible areas of disagreement to find ways of minimising disruptions to each other's controlling.

Keeping an open mind about people's difficulties

We have described some specific examples of conflicts in this chapter. These are presented with the goal of illustrating the kinds of conflicts that people using secondary care mental health services might report. The key point of taking a PCT approach, however, is not to focus on the content of what we have presented as problems in this chapter (e.g., conflicts over medication, hearing voices, or maintaining contact with mental health services) but for mental health services to create the conditions that will allow any patient, whatever their background or culture, to begin to face, explore, and resolve the difficulties that they want to focus on. In fact, there is no need for the services to be fully aware of what these are for each person, but rather, from the outside, to creatively provide environments, settings, resources, and social interactions that enable patients to regain control of what matters to them in their lives. Getting regular feedback and suggestions from patients themselves will be critical to the development of services, with patients as equal, or even more influential, than the staff themselves on suggesting and evaluating these ideas. Those practitioners who are willing to keep an open mind about the nature of people's difficulties, and who approach the exploration of these problems with a genuine sense of curiosity, are likely to be experienced as most helpful by patients (Griffiths, Mansell, Edge, & Tai, 2019; Griffiths, Mansell, Edge, Carey, et al., 2019).

Conclusions

In this chapter, we have endeavoured to set out how PCT principles might inform the design and delivery of mental health services. We have argued that health and mental health can be understood as states where people are able to maintain effective control over aspects of their experience that they value. Loss of control is associated with distress. Rather than aiming to treat diagnosable disorders or to reduce symptoms, the aim of services should instead be to promote individuals' controlling, and alleviate psychological distress as defined by the person seeking support. One of the key sources of distress for people using mental health services is internal conflict because it disrupts the process of control. As such, services and practitioners should be oriented towards helping people resolve distressing conflicts. This can be achieved by creating opportunities for people to explore their problems in depth, by keeping an open mind about the nature of people's problems, and by fostering an environment where people feel able to express themselves openly. Through this approach, people using mental health services can develop new and less distressing perspectives on their problems. Through understanding people as controllers, we can design mental health services that are potentially more helpful and humane, and that use limited resources more efficiently.

References

Allsopp, K., Read, J., Corcoran, R., & Kinderman, P. (2019). Heterogeneity in psychiatric diagnostic classification. *Psychiatry Research*, *279*, 15–22. https://doi.org/10.1016/j.psychres.2019.07.005

American Psychiatric Association. (2013). *Diagnostic and statistical manual of mental disorders* (5th ed.). https://dsm.psychiatryonline.org/doi/book/10.1176/appi.books.9780890425596

Bäuml, J., Froböse, T., Kraemer, S., Rentrop, M., & Pitschel-Walz, G. (2006). Psychoeducation: A basic psychotherapeutic intervention for patients with schizophrenia and their families. *Schizophrenia Bulletin*, *32*(SUPPL.1), S1–S9. https://doi.org/10.1093/schbul/sbl017

Billman, G. E. (2020). Homeostasis: The underappreciated and far too often ignored central organizing principle of physiology. In *Frontiers in Physiology* (Vol. 11). www.frontiersin.org/articles/10.3389/fphys.2020.00200

Carey, T. A. (2006). *The Method of Levels: How to do psychotherapy without getting in the way*. Living Control Systems Publishing.

Carey, T. A. (2008a). Conflict, as the Achilles heel of perceptual control, offers a unifying approach to the formulation of psychological problems. *Counselling Psychology Review*, *23*(4), 5–16. http://psycnet.apa.org/record/2009-03454-003

Carey, T. A. (2008b). Perceptual Control Theory and the Method of Levels: Further contributions to a transdiagnostic perspective. *International Journal of Cognitive Therapy*, *1*(3), 237–255. https://doi.org/10.1521/ijct.2008.1.3.237

Carey, T. A. (2016). Health is control. *Annals of Behavioural Science*, *2*(13), 1–3. http://behaviouralscience.imedpub.com/behavioural-science-psycology/health-is-control.pdf

Carey, T. A. (2017). *Patient-perspective care: A new paradigm for health systems and services* (1st ed.). Routledge.

Carey, T. A., Tai, S. J., & Stiles, W. B. (2013). Effective and efficient: Using patient-led appointment scheduling in routine mental health practice in remote Australia. *Professional Psychology: Research & Practice*, *44*(6), 405–414. https://doi.org/10.1037/a0035038

Claassen, D., & Priebe, S. (2007). Ethical aspects of assertive outreach. *Psychiatry*, *6*(2), 45–48. https://doi.org/10.1016/j.mppsy.2006.11.007

Galderisi, S., Heinz, A., Kastrup, M., Beezhold, J., & Sartorius, N. (2015). Toward a new definition of mental health. *World Psychiatry*, *14*(2), 231–233. https://doi.org/10.1002/wps.20231

García-Pérez, L., Linertová, R., Serrano-Pérez, P., Trujillo-Martín, M., Rodríguez-Rodríguez, L., Valcárcel-Nazco, C., & Del Pino-Sedeño, T. (2020). Interventions to improve medication adherence in mental health: the update of a systematic review of cost-effectiveness. *International Journal of Psychiatry in Clinical Practice*, *24*(4), 416–427. https://doi.org/10.1080/13651501.2020.1782434

Greenwood, K. E., Sweeney, A., Williams, S., Garety, P., Kuipers, E., Scott, J., & Peters, E. (2010). CHoice of Outcome In Cbt for psychosEs (CHOICE): The development of a new service user-led outcome measure of CBT for psychosis. *Schizophrenia Bulletin*, *36*(1), 126–135. https://doi.org/10.1093/schbul/sbp117

Griffiths, R., & Carey, T. A. (2020). Advancing nursing practice for improved health outcomes using the principles of perceptual control theory. *Nursing Philosophy*, February, 1–8. https://doi.org/10.1111/nup.12301

Griffiths, R., Mansell, W., Edge, D., Carey, T. A., Peel, H., & Tai, S.J. (2019a). 'It was me answering my own questions': Experiences of method of levels therapy amongst people with first-episode psychosis. *International Journal of Mental Health Nursing*, *28*(3), 1–14. https://doi.org/10.1111/inm.12576

Griffiths, R., Mansell, W., Edge, D., & Tai, S. (2019b). Sources of distress in first-episode psychosis: A systematic review and qualitative metasynthesis. *Qualitative Health Research*, *29*(1), 107–123. https://doi.org/10.1177/1049732318790544

Hower, K. I., Vennedey, V., Hillen, H. A., Kuntz, L., Stock, S., Pfaff, H., & Ansmann, L. (2019). Implementation of patient-centred care: Which organisational determinants matter from decision maker's perspective? Results from a qualitative interview study across various health and social care organisations. *BMJ Open*, *9*(4), e027591. https://doi.org/10.1136/bmjopen-2018-027591

Huber, M., André Knottnerus, J., Green, L., Van Der Horst, H., Jadad, A. R., Kromhout, D., Leonard, B., Lorig, K., Loureiro, M. I., Van Der Meer, J. W. M., Schnabel, P., Smith, R., Van Weel, C., & Smid, H. (2011). How should we define health? *British Medcal Journal (Online)*, *343*(7817), 1–3. https://doi.org/10.1136/bmj.d4163

Law, H., & Morrison, A. P. (2014). Recovery in psychosis: A delphi study with experts by experience. *Schizophrenia Bulletin*, *40*(6), 1347–1355. https://doi.org/10.1093/schbul/sbu047

Lawrence, C., Jones, J., & Cooper, M. (2010). Hearing voices in a non-psychiatric population. *Behavioural and Cognitive Psychotherapy*, *38*(3), 363–373. https://doi.org/10.1017/S1352465810000172

Maijer, K., Begemann, M. J. H., Palmen, S. J. M. C., Leucht, S., & Sommer, I. E. C. (2018). Auditory hallucinations across the lifespan: A systematic review and meta-analysis. *Psychological Medicine*, *48*(6), 879–888. https://doi.org/10.1017/S0033291717002367

Marken, R. S. (2021). *The study of living control systems: A guide to doing research on purpose*. Cambridge University Press.

Marková, I. S., & Berrios, G. E. (1992). The meaning of insight in clinical psychiatry. *The British Journal of Psychiatry*, *160*, 850–860). Royal College of Psychiatrists. https://doi.org/10.1192/bjp.160.6.850

McCance, T., McCormack, B., & Dewing, J. (2011). An exploration of person-centredness in practice. *Online Journal of Issues in Nursing*, *16*(2), 1.

National Institute for Health and Care Excellence (NICE). (2014). Psychosis and schizophrenia in adults: Prevention and management. In *Nice*. https://doi.org/10.1002/14651858.CD010823.pub2.Copyright

National Institute for Health and Clinical Excellence. (2022). Depression in adults: Treatment and management NICE guideline. *NICE Guideline*, *June*. www.nice.org.uk/guidance/ng222

NHS England, the National Collaborating Centre for Mental Health, & National Institute for Health and Care Excellence. (2016). *Implementing the early intervention in psychosis access and waiting time standard: Guidance* (p. 57). www.england.nhs.uk/mentalhealth/wp-content/uploads/sites/29/2016/04/eip-guidance.pdf

Osatuke, K., Ciesla, J., Kasckow, J. W., Zisook, S., & Mohamed, S. (2008). Insight in schizophrenia: A review of etiological models and supporting research. *Comprehensive Psychiatry*, *49*(1), 70–77. https://doi.org/10.1016/j.comppsych.2007.08.001

Powers, W. T. (1973). *Behavior: The control of perception*. Aldine.

Powers, W. T. (2005). *Behavior: The control of perception* (2nd ed.). Benchmark Publications.

Robinson, J. H., Callister, L. C., Berry, J. A., & Dearing, K. A. (2008). Patient-centered care and adherence: definitions and applications to improve outcomes. *Journal of the American Academy of Nurse Practitioners*, *20*(12), 600–607. https://doi.org/10.1111/j.1745-7599.2008.00360.x

Soltan, M., & Girguis, J. (2017). How to approach the mental state examination. *British Medical Journal (Clinical Research Ed.)*, *357*, j1821. https://doi.org/10.1136/sbmj.j1821

Stiles, W. B., Barkham, M., Connell, J., & Mellor-Clark, J. (2008). Responsive regulation of treatment duration in routine practice in United Kingdom primary care settings: Replication in a larger sample. *Journal of Consulting and Clinical Psychology*, *76*(2), 298–305. https://doi.org/10.1037/0022-006X.76.2.298

Thirioux, B., Harika-Germaneau, G., Langbour, N., & Jaafari, N. (2019). The relation between empathy and insight in psychiatric disorders: Phenomenological, etiological, and neuro-functional mechanisms. *Frontiers in Psychiatry*, *10*, 966. https://doi.org/10.3389/fpsyt.2019.00966

Timimi, S. (2014). No more psychiatric labels: Why formal psychiatric diagnostic systems should be abolished. *International Journal of Clinical and Health Psychology*, *14*(3), 208–215. https://doi.org/10.1016/j.ijchp.2014.03.004

Warwick, H., Mansell, W., Porter, C., & Tai, S. (2019). 'What people diagnosed with bipolar disorder experience as distressing': A meta-synthesis of qualitative research. *Journal of Affective Disorders*, *248*(January), 108–130. https://doi.org/10.1016/j.jad.2019.01.024

Waters, F., & Fernyhough, C. (2017). Hallucinations: A systematic review of points of similarity and difference across diagnostic classes. *Schizophrenia Bulletin*, *43*(1), 32–43. https://doi.org/10.1093/schbul/sbw132

Willett, A. B. S., Marken, R. S., Parker, M. G., & Mansell, W. (2017). Control blindness: Why people can make incorrect inferences about the intentions of others. *Attention, Perception, and Psychophysics*, *79*(3), 841–849. https://doi.org/10.3758/s13414-016-1268-3

World Health Organization. (2018). International classification of diseases for mortality and morbidity statistics (11th Revision). In *World Health Organization* (Vol. 11). https://icd.who.int/browse11/l-m/en

Chapter 4

Individual Psychological Therapy

The Method of Levels

Introduction

In preceding chapters, we have described how Perceptual Control Theory (PCT) can be used to shape the design and delivery of secondary mental healthcare services. Using the principles of PCT, we have argued, it is possible to radically redesign mental health services to make them more effective, efficient, and humane. In addition to providing clear principles that can be used to shape the overall design of mental health services, however, PCT can also be used to guide individual practitioners in their clinical work. An example of this is a talking therapy called the Method of Levels (MOL; Carey, 2006; Carey et al., 2015; Mansell et al., 2013), which is an approach to psychotherapy that directly applies PCT principles.

The purpose of this chapter is to describe the practice of MOL and to clarify exactly how PCT principles inform the approach. We have included a case vignette to illustrate the way in which an MOL conversation might occur. There is also a personal reflection of engaging with MOL, written from the perspective of someone who has experienced an MOL session first-hand. Details of an innovative approach to scheduling therapy appointments that is informed by PCT principles, which we touched on in the previous chapter, are also described in more depth. Throughout the chapter we will highlight why the MOL approach to therapy might be particularly well suited to secondary mental healthcare settings.

Psychological therapy in secondary care

The ambition to offer users of secondary mental healthcare services access to appropriate and timely psychological interventions is not a new endeavour. Efforts to overcome barriers to the implementation of individual and family psychological interventions for people using secondary care go back several decades (e.g., Fadden, 1997; Tarrier et al., 1999). The goal of offering widespread, timely, and effective access to psychological interventions in secondary care, however, remains elusive (e.g., Ince et al., 2015). Given the numerous

DOI: 10.4324/9781003041344-4

policy announcements on this topic, coupled with increased financial investment, and a proliferation of programmes designed to train staff in the delivery of psychological interventions, the lack of progress in this area is dispiriting. A recent UK audit of people using secondary care services seeking psychological therapy for problems with anxiety and depression provided confirmation that these access problems persist (Healthcare Quality Improvement Partnership, 2020). Amongst survey respondents, 41% had to wait more than 18 weeks to access psychological therapy. Even more concerning, 9% of respondents reported waiting one to two years for therapy. One participant summed up these findings with the following quote, which we would endorse:

> If you are acutely unwell to need secondary services, 18 weeks or more is a long time. That is saying nothing of the people who had to wait almost two years.
>
> (Healthcare Quality Improvement Partnership, 2020, p. 15)

Problems in accessing psychological therapy exist even within relatively well resourced secondary care services, such as specialist early intervention in psychosis teams (Royal College of Psychiatrists, 2020).

A PCT perspective on effective psychological therapy

As discussed in Chapter 2, according to PCT, the terms 'health' and 'control' can be considered synonymous (Carey, 2016). The means through which control is achieved and maintained, from this perspective, can be distilled into three core principles. These can be summarised as: control, conflict, and reorganisation. It has been argued that these core principles can be used to inform the delivery of an effective psychological therapy (Carey et al., 2015). We will briefly revisit each of the three principles outlined in Chapter 2, before outlining how they have been directly applied to develop MOL. We will also argue that MOL has the capacity to address many of the practical and theoretical limitations that have restricted access to psychological therapy for users of secondary mental healthcare.

The term control refers to a dynamic process involving the continual adjustment of behaviour in order to maintain perceptions in line with internally specified preferences (known as 'reference values') held for the state of those perceptions (Powers et al., 1960a, 1960b; Powers, 1973, 2005). Most of the time, control is achieved through an apparently effortless process, much of which occurs outside awareness (Powers, 2005). When engaging someone in conversation, for example, perceptions being controlled might include voice volume, physical proximity, the content of the conversation, and the perception of how effectively the points to be conveyed are being communicated. It is unlikely, however, that many of these factors will be held in direct awareness during the process of conversing with another person. The actions taken to effectively maintain these perceptions will need to vary depending on factors such as the environmental conditions where the conversation is taking place and the interests and capacities of the other person. When moving from a quiet corridor to a loud meeting room, for example, in order to make yourself heard, you might increase the volume of your voice relative to the overall change in background noise. Alternatively, you might decrease the volume or your voice if you have another goal of sharing information discreetly. As we saw in Chapter 2, the process of control is so fundamental to human health, it is unsurprising that being unable to effectively control important perceptions results in psychological distress.

While loss of control can occur for a variety of reasons, one common reason amongst people seeking help from mental health services is that they are in a state of conflict (Carey, 2008). As with other concepts arising from PCT, the theory offers a very precise definition of the term conflict. Conflict is said to occur in situations where people hold two or more incompatible reference values for the state of the same perception (Powers, 2005). If a person wants to take their child to school, but they are overwhelmed by a sense that others mean to harm them whenever they leave the house, they are experiencing a conflict. Not leaving the house would mean that the person is unable to take their child to school. Leaving the house would mean feeling vulnerable to harm from others. Attempts to meet either one of these goals, therefore, actively disrupt efforts to achieve the other. An effective psychological therapy, from a PCT perspective, is one that supports people to resolve the underlying conflicts that are maintaining their distress (Carey et al., 2015; Carey, 2011).

The way that people resolve conflicts, PCT proposes, is through a trial-and-error system called reorganisation (Marken & Powers, 1989; Powers, 2005). Here, random changes are introduced to the controlling of the individual. Changes will persist when they have the effect of reducing the gap between a person's current perceptions and their preferences for the state of those perceptions. If the change does not have the effect of reducing this discrepancy, before too long, another random change will be introduced into the system. This process continues until the differences between current and desired perceptions are reduced to a level deemed satisfactory (Marken & Carey, 2015b). It is this process of reorganisation that is believed to enable people to resolve the conflicts that are disrupting control and maintaining distress (Carey, 2011).

The Method of Levels

The Method of Levels (MOL) aims to directly apply the three principles described above – control, conflict, and reorganisation – to the practice of psychotherapy. The result is a talking therapy that can be applied flexibly across a diverse range of clinical contexts.

Often described as a transdiagnostic cognitive therapy, in reality, the term 'adiagnostic' more accurately captures the MOL approach to psychotherapy.

The term transdiagnostic implies that a therapy is applicable to the difficulties of people whose problems fall across a variety of different diagnostic categories. A therapy that is described as adiagnostic, on the other hand, suggests that whether or not a person has received a particular diagnosis is entirely inconsequential as to how the therapy is delivered. Irrespective of whether a person has received multiple diagnoses, or none at all, the principles that inform the delivery of MOL remain the same.

Focusing on distress not symptoms

Many talking therapies are designed with the aim of reducing symptoms or syndromes (groups of apparently related symptoms), which are believed to be the result of specific disorders. In the case of people experiencing psychosis-related difficulties, for example, the Positive and Negative Syndrome Scale (PANSS; Kay et al., 1987) is often used as a measure of a particular intervention's effectiveness. If someone's symptoms reduce, as measured by this scale, the intervention is deemed to have been successful. It is notable that nearly all randomised controlled trials of cognitive behaviour therapy (CBT) for psychosis use symptom reduction as the primary outcome measure (Greenwood et al., 2010). This focus on symptom reduction is not limited to psychological interventions for psychosis. Similar symptom measures are commonly used to evaluate outcomes for people reporting depression (Beck et al., 1996), anxiety (Spitzer et al., 2006), trauma (Weiss & Marmar, 1997), and a range of other problems identified as mental health disorders.

Therapists delivering MOL, however, are not aiming to reduce symptoms or treat diagnosable disorders. The Oxford English Dictionary offers the following definition of a symptom: 'a sign or indication *of* something' (Oxford University Press, n.d., para. 2). The something referred to in this definition, from the perspective of PCT, is the presence of a conflict. Specific symptoms might represent a useful starting point from which somebody might begin to explore their difficulties. From a PCT point of view, talking therapies that remain focused at the symptom level, however, will be unlikely to resolve underlying conflicts directly and effectively. When goal conflicts are resolved during engagement with a psychological therapy aimed at treating symptoms, it would be considered that the resolution occurred serendipitously rather than by design. MOL is a therapeutic procedure that addresses goal conflict directly (Carey et al., 2015; Carey & Mullan, 2008; Mansell et al., 2013).

In contrast to approaches that aim to reduce symptoms, MOL is designed to reduce psychological distress (Carey, 2009; Carey et al., 2015). This is because the behaviours, thoughts, and emotions that might ordinarily be identified as symptoms of mental health disorders are not inherently and necessarily distressing. The experience of hearing voices that others cannot is a useful example of this point. Hearing voices is an experience that is frequently identified as a symptom of a mental health disorder and subsequently targeted by mental health services, both through the use of medications and psychosocial interventions. There is good evidence, however, that large numbers of people regularly hear voices without this experience causing significant distress or disruption to their lives (Beavan et al., 2011). In fact, many people actually report that hearing voices is a positive, meaningful, or helpful experience (Valavanis et al., 2019). In our experience, people seeking help from mental health services who report problematic voice hearing are generally doing so because of the impact this has on other areas of their life. Someone might worry, for example, about the way in which their voice hearing experiences will be perceived by others. Alternatively, they might have concerns that hearing voices will impair their ability to form meaningful relationships with others. Or perhaps the content of the voice itself is unacceptable to them because it conflicts with other important goals. A person might hear a voice, for example, that is instructing them to harm others. If harming others, however, is at odds with deeply held beliefs about non-violence this will establish a conflict situation for the individual which will result in distress. Similarly, the voice they hear might instruct them to harm, or even kill, themselves, yet they might want to live a pain free life. This conflict could also be expected to generate significant distress for the person. From a PCT perspective, voice hearing is likely to be problematic only when it creates the kinds of conflicts for the person that we have illustrated here. The view of voice hearing as distressing that we are offering here is supported by evidence that the content of individuals' voice hearing is often thematically linked to their personal goals (Varese et al., 2016). Where a conflict exists between voice content and a person's valued goals, this is likely to be distressing. The idea that symptoms are a source of distress when they are associated with conflicts applies equally to symptoms of other so-called disorders, such as anxiety or depression. Symptoms such as loss of motivation or feeling anxious, for example, generally create distress when they interfere with activities that are valued by the person, such as working, socialising, or caring for one's children. In fact, it could even be that the symptoms of loss of motivation or anxiety are manifestations of conflicts: staying at work and earning a wage versus resigning and finding more meaningful work; or socialising with new friends versus not risking rejection; or caring for one's children versus escaping responsibilities and having fun.

Treating people as individuals

When taking a PCT perspective, it is apparent that people have a plethora of preferred experiences that differ from one person to the next, and this is the case over a wide range of experiential levels (Powers, 2008; Runkel, 2003). The levels of experience range from the sensory experiences each person finds comforting and the various unpleasant feelings they try not to experience, right up to the kinds of principles each person seeks to uphold in their everyday life, and the kind of person they want to be. Each of us changes our actions in the current moment to achieve and maintain our own, idiosyncratic, preferred experiences. So, as clinicians, we have to respect not only the individuality of every person, but also that we cannot assume that behaviours we observe are the same behaviours from one person to another or even with the same person in different situations. Behaviour as it is observed from a third-person perspective is a different phenomenon from the way it is experienced from a first-person perspective (Carey, 2017). PCT, therefore, explains the necessity of treating each person as an individual, and maintaining an attitude of openness and optimism regarding the change that, ideally, will occur in therapy. With an understanding of PCT principles, MOL therapists optimistically assume that change will happen even if it doesn't happen in the time frame or in the way that might be expected in other therapeutic approaches (Carey et al., 2015; Marken & Carey, 2015b).

Furthermore, understanding therapeutic change as being the result of the reorganisation of higher-level goals has important implications for how psychological therapy should be delivered. As discussed, the reorganisation system is believed to be a random process that relies on introducing changes into a control system on a trial-and-error basis (Marken & Powers, 1989; Powers, 2005). Consequently, it is not possible to predict exactly how long it will take someone to experience the changes they want. Some people will experience helpful changes relatively quickly. For other people, however, the process of change will take a longer period of time. So, the PCT clinician will have an open mind as to the rate of change for any particular individual (Carey et al., 2015). This openminded attitude can convey hope that even the most longstanding problems can be overcome, as well as an appreciation that some patients can find genuinely effective solutions to their difficulties very quickly. It might also occur that, sometimes, things seem to get worse before they get better as reorganisation produces one potential solution after another (Carey, 2011).

Putting patients in control

What would an effective therapy look like if we were to adopt PCT principles? It would be flexible, distress-focused, and patient-led with regard to the content of therapy conversations and the booking of therapy appointments. Indeed, the patient should be able to control whatever parameter of the therapy they desire (location, tone of voice, comfortable seating distance), within the constraints of the resources of the service, and without interfering with what the therapist, and other people, need to control.

The issue of who decides when and how people access psychological therapy is an important one. Given that access to psychotherapy is a finite resource, many secondary care services conduct some form of screening process to determine which patients are likely to derive the most benefit from engaging with a talking therapy. Whether therapy actually needs to be rationed in this way is a question we will consider separately. For now, we will consider another issue: who is best placed to make judgements about who should receive therapy (Carey, 2005)? A recent UK report into the capacity of secondary mental services to deliver psychological therapy for people reporting anxiety and depression contains revealing comments about how the rationing of therapy is taking place (Healthcare Quality Improvement Partnership, 2020). For example, one patient stated:

> I waited over twelve months to even get an appointment with a therapist, and when I did get one they decided I was 'too well' for therapy.
>
> (Healthcare Quality Improvement Partnership, 2020, p. 15)

In addition to this individual's prolonged wait to be considered for a talking therapy, which is concerning in itself, the above quote illustrates something else. It is an example of how patients' preferences regarding the support they would prefer are often considered secondary to clinicians' views on this matter. In this case, the clinician's judgement was that the person's problems were insufficiently severe to justify access to a talking therapy. This perspective was prioritised above the patient's demonstrated commitment to engage with therapy by waiting a year to be offered an appointment. From a PCT perspective, the person seeking help is best placed to determine whether or not they could benefit from access to a talking therapy (Carey, 2017). Where clinicians are making decisions about the severity of peoples' problems and their suitability for psychological therapy, it should be acknowledged that they are doing so from their own perspective (Carey, 2017). This is the case whether a clinician's decision is guided by pragmatic or resource issues, or their 'clinical judgement' about what is in the best interests of the patient.

In the well-known folk tale, Goldilocks tasted the three bears' bowls of porridge before deciding that each was either 'too hot', 'too cold', or 'just right'. Prioritising the perspective of clinicians over patients on the issue of when people should access therapy is akin to Goldilocks being told which bowl of porridge is right for her by someone who has not tasted any of them. Crucially, even if someone else did taste them, they could never know what was 'too hot' or 'just right' from Goldilocks's perspective. Currently, in secondary care services it appears to be the case that many decisions regarding what will be 'just right' for patients are made by people other than the patients. People assuming that they know what is best for others, and then acting on that assumption, is, from a PCT perspective, at the core of many of our social problems (Marken & Carey, 2015a).

The Method of Levels in practice

So, how would a Method of Levels (MOL) conversation actually occur? Practitioners more familiar with other psychological therapies might be surprised to learn that delivering MOL requires therapists to adopt just two goals (Carey,

2006). The simplicity of the MOL approach can contrast starkly with guidelines for the delivery of other psychological therapies. Many therapies, for example, require practitioners to learn a wide range of tools and techniques, and know when to apply each of these appropriately at different stages of therapy. There can also be an expectation that the therapist will need to become familiar with variants of the therapy that can be applied to patients with different presenting problems or across different contexts. This might mean learning about a variety of conceptual models specific to different disorders and how these inform the process of formulating patients' difficulties. In contrast, practitioners delivering MOL are required to pursue the same two goals, irrespective of the nature of the patient's specific problems or the context in which the therapist is working.

The simplicity of the two goals of MOL, however, does not necessarily mean that MOL is easier to learn or deliver than other therapies – in our experience, becoming proficient in MOL requires practice and hard work on behalf of the therapist. MOL could be considered simple but not easy. Learning the two goals of MOL is rarely the main challenge for practitioners new to this approach. What can often be more difficult, in our experience, is not doing all the things that might be quite routine in other therapies but that will obstruct the two goals of MOL. People often feel compelled, for example, to give patients advice or offer reassurance. While a therapist might engage in these behaviours with the best of intentions, the aim of MOL is to help people develop their own novel perspectives on problems. Advice and reassurance, offered from the perspective of the therapist, is likely to be irrelevant or distracting (Carey et al., 2015). Potentially, this could even prevent the patient from generating their own solutions to distressing problems. Practitioners new to MOL might also struggle to avoid making assumptions about a patient's current experiences, for example by making statements such as, 'That must be very difficult'. Whilst the experience the patient is describing might indeed be very difficult, the MOL approach is one founded on remaining curious and enquiring. Statements based on assumptions miss valuable opportunities to help the patient explore and resolve their difficulties. So now that we have considered what MOL does not involve, let us focus instead on what actually does happen during an MOL session.

Goal 1: Encourage the person to talk freely about a problem

The first goal for therapists aiming to deliver MOL is to encourage patients to speak openly about a problem that they are willing to discuss (Carey, 2006). The therapist is aiming to create the conditions necessary for the patient to speak about whatever is on their mind, ideally without filtering or screening the content of their speech prior to its expression (Carey et al., 2012). Clearly, the specific conditions that one patient perceives to be right for them will not be helpful, or 'just right', for other patients. Some patients will attend MOL sessions feeling very ready to talk about what is troubling them and the therapist will be required to do very little to encourage them to discuss their problems. Other patients, however, might feel very reticent about attending a therapy session, and it might take some time for them to feel safe enough to express whatever it is that is bothering them. For this reason, although the principles underpinning a therapist's conduct remain the same, the way they go about this might vary significantly between sessions. Therapists, for example, might be required to be very active in sessions when working with a patient whose mood appears elevated. If the patient is speaking quickly, or rapidly moving between topics of conversation, the therapist's job will be to try and keep up with what the patient is expressing. If, however, a patient seems withdrawn, subdued, suspicious of the therapist, or is struggling to concentrate, the therapist will have to adjust their approach accordingly.

Goal 2: Ask about disruptions

The second goal for therapists who are aiming to deliver MOL is to ask the patient about what are called 'disruptions' (Carey, 2006). These are indications that the person's awareness has momentarily shifted from the current topic of conversation onto another aspect of their experience. In these situations, the person's awareness will often settle on internal experiences relevant to the problem being described. There are a wide range of potential changes that could indicate the presence of a disruption. These might include hesitating, emphasising, or stumbling over particular words, changes in body posture or facial expression, or apparent changes in affect. Patients might laugh at something they just said, pause, and briefly seem to lose their train of thought, shift uncomfortably in their seat, or become tearful for a few seconds. The therapist's job when a potential disruption is noticed, is simply to ask about it. Questions such as 'What crossed your mind just then?', or 'Is something else occurring to you while we're talking?' can help the person capture fleeting shifts in awareness that would otherwise go unnoticed. The purpose in asking about disruptions is to help the person shift their awareness to ever higher levels within the perceptual hierarchy until they reach the point of the conflict that is creating the distress (Carey, 2008; Carey et al., 2015). In fact, more accurately, the person's awareness will need to go beyond this point to a level above the conflicted control systems; to the place in the hierarchy from where the incompatible reference signals are set. With the PCT assumption that reorganisation follows awareness, MOL therapists consider that if they can help patients talk about ideas and beliefs that seem to be above or 'meta' to the conflict, then this is the place where reorganisation will occur (Carey et al., 2015; Marken & Carey, 2015b). If patients remained focused on their symptoms, reorganisation will stay at the symptom level. Reorganising symptoms, however, is not likely to have any lasting effect on the conflict. It is the process of directing awareness, and therefore reorganisation, to levels above the conflict that enables people to resolve conflicts that are creating their distress (Carey, 2011; Carey et al., 2015). If, after asking about a disruption, the patient discovers a topic of discussion that it would be useful to explore further, the therapist then switches back to the first goal of MOL by encouraging the person to keep talking about the new topic. Sessions of MOL continue in this iterative fashion until either the patient decides that further discussion is not necessary at this point, or the therapist needs to end the session for practical reasons, such as time constraints.

Case vignette to illustrate the Method of Levels in action

The following case vignette illustrates MOL occurring. The fictitious patient is an amalgam of real secondary care patients who have received MOL.

Ray was a 53-year-old man who had been working as an NHS manager up until the onset of an episode of mania involving psychotic experiences that occurred several months after he had been promoted to a highly challenging role in the organisation. He was brought into hospital after attempting to jump from his 14th floor apartment window. He had become convinced that he was a negative influence on the world and would contaminate everyone with whom he came into contact. Ray had eventually recovered from his episode after two months on psychiatric wards, and he was being seen in an outpatient service. He started by requesting sessions on a weekly basis, but gradually he reduced this to monthly, having around 15 MOL sessions in total, each between 30 and 60 minutes. This vignette is from one of the early sessions.

Vignette 4.1 Method of Levels case vignette

[initial greetings and completion of a brief measure – the Outcome Rating Scale (Miller et al., 2003)]

Sarah (Therapist): So, what do you want to talk about today, Ray?

Ray: I've been writing about my time in hospital again and brought what I've written to show you.

Sarah: OK, thanks [Ray hands two handwritten pages to Sarah]. Do you want me to read this now, or would you rather talk about it, or something else?

Ray: Mmmm. Could you read it after this session? I've got some other things I wanted to talk about.

Sarah: OK, of course, I can read this. Is there anything you particularly want from me after I have read it?

Ray: Not really. I just want to keep a record of it all. It helps to get it out of my mind and onto the page.

Sarah: Yes, of course. So, do you want to talk about getting things out of your mind, or the other things you mentioned?

Ray: Well, I think they are all related actually.

Sarah: Could you tell me how?

Ray: Well, I just get really obsessed by what happened to me. I get stuck in a daze. Sometimes an hour has gone past, and I haven't done anything. That's the problem.

Sarah: Tell me how it is a problem again?

Ray: I want to get into a routine and do things I enjoy doing. I know that will keep me well, along with taking my medication. But I just get stuck … in this daze.

Sarah: How dazed do you feel right now?

Ray: I feel OK at the moment I think because I have just written what was in my head and it is out of my head for a while.

Sarah: What's left in your head right now?

Ray: It's clear. It's just thoughts about other things, which feels good.

Sarah: So, when you are 'dazed' – what's going on then?

Ray: I think about everything that happened to me in hospital, but it's a jumble. When I write it down for you, I am trying to put it all together in the right order, so it makes sense to me. And so I can explain what happened to other people.

Sarah: Can you tell me how you think this will help?

Ray: If I can understand what happened to me, step by step, then I can stop it happening again. I don't want to ruin my relationships. I am so lucky to have a partner who came through this with me and is still here. But I also want to get well enough so that I can work again. And I can't see that happening yet.

Sarah: What can you see happening?

Ray: I can see myself getting so stressed again that I have another episode [looks tearful].

Sarah: What's going on for you there?

Ray: I was just thinking of the moment that I decided to take on this promotion. I know it was too much. My father had just died. I knew the department was already falling apart. But I just powered head on into it.

Sarah: Head on?

Ray: Yes, I was determined that I could do it.

Sarah: What's that about? Your determination?

Ray: Whenever I put my mind to something, I do it. But I do it whatever the consequences.

Sarah: [interrupts] Are you thinking of the consequences just there?

Ray: Well [laughs] this time the consequences were extreme!
Sarah: What did you think as you laughed just then?
Ray: Well, it's just like what's happening now. I get obsessed by solving something, by doing it all perfectly, methodically. But at the same time – I haven't sat down with my partner for a week. I haven't been out in the garden. I haven't phoned my brother.
Sarah: How are all those things weighing up for you as you talk about them?
Ray: Well, look. I've got to get well, and I've got to approach this in the right way. But I've also got to keep my everyday life going – or I'll lose everything again …
Sarah: [interrupts] So how are they both looking to you right now?
Ray: They are looking like they are both important. Actually, they are both vital.
Sarah: [interrupts] Exactly the same importance?
Ray: [pauses and looks to the side]
Sarah: What's going on right now?
Ray: I'm imagining writing down my hospital experiences in the morning, when they are fresh in my mind, and I am then thinking about sorting out the greenhouse as the weather is nice. And I'm thinking about phoning my brother.
Sarah: How is that unfolding right now?
Ray: It's making me think that I can do both. I just need to be able to switch off and do something.
Sarah: How do you switch off?
Ray: That's what I can't do.
Sarah: Ever?
Ray: Well, it must happen. I'm switched off now.
Sarah: What do you think is letting you do it now?
Ray: It's about talking openly with you, so when I get something bothering me in my head, I can let it out. Normally, I just keep one worry after another swimming around.
Sarah: How fast do they swim?
Ray: Too fast to concentrate on doing something more useful, and too fast to focus. When I talk them through, they swim slower, until it's nearly still.
Sarah: How still do you want your mind to be?
Ray: Actually, I don't mind my mind being fast as long as I can control it. So maybe it's not the speed that's the problem, but when it's really fast it's hard to control.
Sarah: So how much control do you want over how fast your worries are?

Ray: I think I need to be in control of them. I feel in control now.
Sarah: So complete control?
Ray: Nearly, enough to focus, like now. Phew!
Sarah: What's the 'phew' about?
Ray: I feel like I've talked a lot. I've got something to think about after this. I'm not sure I've got much more to say at the moment. I feel a bit tired, but it's been really useful today.
Sarah: OK. Anything else you'd like to tell me about what was helpful, or not today?
Ray: It all seemed helpful, letting me work things out for myself.
Sarah: So, no way you want it different?
Ray: No, just like this seems to work for me.
Sarah: OK. Do you want to leave it there then? Or anything else?
Ray: That's all from me today. If I bring something else I've written next time, is that OK?
Sarah: Of course. Do you just want to book a session when you are ready?
Ray: Yes, I'll do that.
Sarah: That's fine then.
Ray: OK.

This session is very typical, although, of course, MOL sessions can be more challenging than this. We chose a relatively straightforward session to make the general principles apparent. First, it should be clear that this session is patient-led. You might have noticed that at the start of the session there were many possible avenues for the conversation. The therapist handled this by remaining open, listening carefully to each of the potential pathways, and trying her best to help Ray choose between them. Then, it appeared that after some questioning Ray chose a path – one that actually drew connections between the different topics he could have talked about. This does not always happen, but it does illustrate that the therapist can help the patient to make the choice without any guidance, advice, or suggestions. The therapist is highly attentive, tracking what Ray is saying, and is piqued by curiosity, frequently asking curious questions about the problem that Ray is describing. Many of these questions are focused on what is occurring for the patient 'right now'. This point might be another significant departure from other therapies that, perhaps, focus instead on memories from the patient's recent or distant past or plans the patient might be imagining for the near or distant future. In MOL, it is assumed that the most direct way to address distress is by examining and exploring it as it occurs, not by remembering it or imagining it (Carey et al., 2015). MOL therapists will definitely ask about the past or the future if it seems appropriate and relevant; however, the focus for the therapist is always about what is happening right now

Reflection 4.1 Stuart's experience of MOL

The whole process felt gentle and exploratory, almost like a dance between me and the therapist. It didn't feel forced at all. Whenever I said something, the therapist would ask a question with real curiosity, and this would make me think again about what I'd said but from a different perspective. It felt like I was leading the therapist around an environment that we were both exploring together. The session came with strong physical and emotional sensations. There were times, for example, when I felt almost tearful during the session. It took me to places that were unexpected, but this was helpful. It led to a good connection between me and the therapist – it felt like they were on my side and interested in what I was saying. I felt like the master of my own destiny during the conversation.

for the patient as they remember or imagine the topic that is currently in their awareness. In the transcript above, many of the questions were used to keep prompting Ray to explore what he was talking about, in order to sustain his awareness on the problem. Some of the questions were about the disruptions – the pauses, uses of certain words, laughs, tears – that spontaneously emerged.

In Reflection 4.1, Stuart discusses his experience of engaging with MOL.

Patient-led scheduling

Patient-led scheduling is an innovative approach to delivering psychological therapy that places the patient in control of the support they receive (Carey, 2017; Carey et al., 2013). As with MOL itself, this approach to appointment scheduling is directly informed by the principles of PCT. Based on an understanding of reorganisation, it is assumed that change in psychological therapy occurs in ways that are unique to the individual, and change can happen at any time (Carey, 2011). It makes sense, therefore, to work from an assumption that different patients will need different numbers and frequencies of sessions in order to get to the point where they have made the changes they want.

The conventional approach to offering therapy is that the service or clinician dictates how many sessions people are offered. Sometimes these decisions are based on the recommendations of published clinical guidelines (e.g., National Institute for Health and Care Excellence (NICE), 2014). At other times, however, the exact reasons for a patient being offered a specific number of sessions can be hard to discern; with the scientific or theoretical rationale behind these decisions remaining opaque. Even in situations where session numbers and therapy duration are dictated by clinical guidelines, it often remains unclear how the authors of those guidelines arrived at that specific number or length of time as being the most appropriate. The consequence of configuring services along these lines, however, is that there is little room for variation between patients. It also fails to emphasise the importance of promoting patient choice and control over the support they receive. The following quote from a recent UK audit illustrates some of the difficulties created by highly protocolised or clinician-led approaches to the delivery of psychological therapy:

> I like the therapy but the sessions were not enough. I feel I need more sessions.
> (Healthcare Quality Improvement Partnership, 2020, p. 17)

Despite the patient reporting that they found the sessions helpful, they were denied the opportunity to engage with this resource for what they perceived to be a sufficient amount of time. This quote contrasts starkly with the findings of our research, which shows that patients really value the control over therapy attendance that the patient-led approach provides (Griffiths, Mansell, Edge, Carey et al., 2019). One participant in the study offered the following description of their experience of patient-led scheduling:

> And I think what was nice about this was, it was very open. You had lots of … you had all these months, and you could come and go as you pleased, and that flexibility was really good.
> (Griffiths et al., 2019, p. 7)

Patient-led appointment scheduling in practice

We have delivered MOL using patient-led appointment scheduling in a range of secondary care settings, including psychiatric inpatient units, early intervention in psychosis services, and mental health outpatient clinics (e.g., Carey et al., 2013; Griffiths, Mansell, Carey, et al., 2019; Jenkins et al., 2020). The exact arrangements needed to establish these systems have differed between settings somewhat, depending on factors such as the resources available and the specific aims of the service. Irrespective of the setting, however, the principles that underpin the arrangements for patient-led scheduling have remained the same. Where possible we maximise the control that patients have over the frequency and duration of sessions, how they go about booking appointments, and decisions about when to stop attending therapy.

We conducted a study to investigate the use of MOL and patient-led scheduling in an early intervention in psychosis service based in a city in Northwest England (Griffiths, Mansell, Carey, et al., 2019). To illustrate how patient-led scheduling works in secondary care, and how patients engage with the system when they have access to it, we are going to explore this study in some detail. Unlike many psychological therapy studies that set pre-specified and, in our view, arbitrary targets for how many therapy sessions participants should receive, we took the decision to make sessions available for a period of ten months. A time period of ten months is also, in many ways, an arbitrary decision. In this case, however, it was largely driven by pragmatic considerations: this was the longest period of time we could offer within the financial and practical constraints of the research project. Ideally, from a PCT perspective, sessions should be accessible whenever a patient decides that it would be useful to attend one. This is an example of the kind of compromises that sometimes have to be made in order to reconcile pragmatic and theoretical imperatives (Carey, 2010). Still, even within the constraints of this study, we were able to give participants significantly more control over how and when they accessed therapy than is possible in standard services.

Participants who were allocated to receive access to MOL sessions were given detailed information about what the therapy involved, how they could book sessions, where they were held, and the length of time that therapy would be available. To increase the chances that participants could find a method of booking a session that was right for them, they could do this either by phoning, texting, or emailing a member of the study team to check session availability and book a session. Alternatively, participants could use an online booking system that enabled them to see all the available appointment slots and select the one that was convenient for them.

Once participants were provided with details that outlined how to book and attend sessions, they were left to make their own decisions about accessing therapy. We did not try to encourage or cajole people into coming along to sessions. Nor did we try to 'assertively outreach' or 'engage' people in therapy. A wonderful feature of the patient-led approach, from our perspective, is that it is supremely respectful of peoples' choices regarding when they think therapy will be helpful and when it is not required. This approach is consistent with many codes of professional practice for healthcare professionals, which advocate being respectful of peoples' right to refuse or withdraw from treatment (e.g., British Psychological Society, 2009; Nursing and Midwifery Council, 2015). For this approach to work, the crucial thing is that people know how to book a session should they need one.

We looked at MOL attendance rates over the course of study to try and understand more about how people make use of therapy sessions when they have the freedom to book them as they wish. Figure 4.1 shows attendance rates for individual participants in the study, with each dot representing an attended MOL session. One striking feature of these data is how dissimilar patterns of attendance are between participants. Some people began attending sessions as soon as the treatment window opened; others waited several weeks or even months before attending their first session. Some people attended MOL sessions fairly regularly in the first weeks before their rates of attendance dropped off. Others, however, preferred to attend more sporadically across the course of the 10-month treatment window. The actual number of sessions that people attended also varied substantially, ranging from zero to ten sessions (n.b., Figure 4.1 only shows attendance rates for participants who booked at least one session).

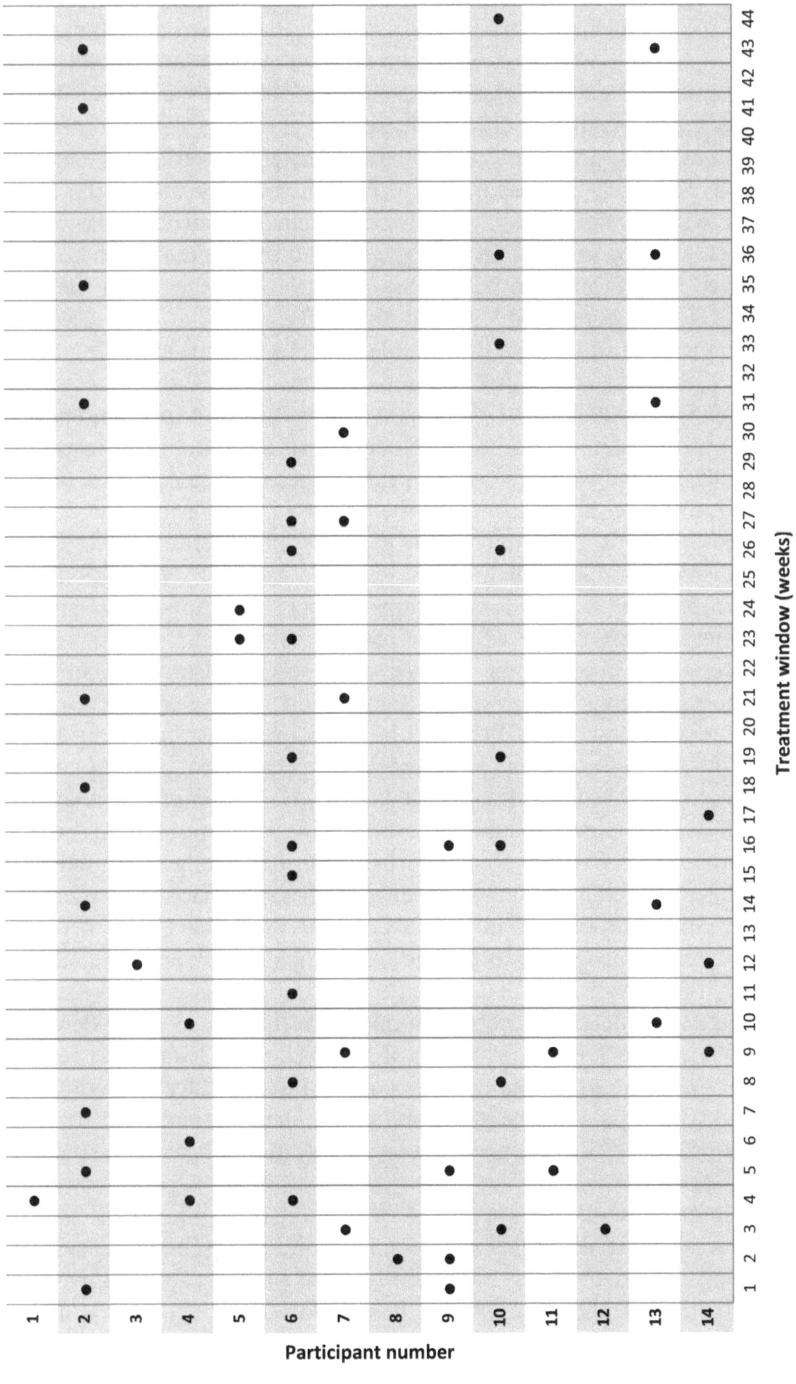

Figure 4.1 Participant MOL session attendance figures for Griffiths et al., (2019). Each dot represents an MOL session booked and attended across the 44-week treatment window.

Before we began this study, we talked to clinicians working in early intervention services about our plans. During these conversations, two main concerns were raised repeatedly. The first was that using a patient-led approach to appointment scheduling would create a demand for therapy that we would be unable to meet. Participants would simply book every available appointment, so the argument went, and there would be insufficient therapist capacity to meet demand. Strangely, the second concern was the opposite of the first. Namely, that without the use of 'assertive engagement', participants would attend very few therapy sessions. In reality, we found that neither of these predictions proved accurate. When people have control over their own therapy appointments, it has been demonstrated to be the case that they use this resource responsibly and in ways that enable them to balance attending therapy sessions with other competing demands (Carey, 2005; Carey & Mullan, 2007; Carey & Spratt, 2009). One participant, for example, stopped attending therapy sessions for a few weeks because their housing situation was insecure, and, quite understandably, resolving this problem became their priority (Griffiths, Mansell, Carey, et al., 2019). Once the housing issue was dealt with, the participant resumed his attendance at therapy sessions. Because each MOL session is a discrete problem-solving exercise, large gaps between sessions do not prove disruptive to the process of therapy. Patients are simply able to attend sessions whenever they decide it will be helpful.

It is interesting to reflect on the ways in which services using conventional approaches to scheduling therapy appointments might have responded to the patterns of therapy attendance displayed by participants in this study. Most participants, for example, waited several weeks after the initial opening of the treatment window before they attended their first MOL appointment. Participant 5 actually waited almost six months to attend his first appointment (before attending two sessions in a fortnight). Perhaps conventionally organised services would have worked hard to try and 'engage' these participants in therapy. It seems more likely, however, that the participants would have been deemed not ready, unwilling, or unable to engage with a talking therapy, and subsequently discharged. We found that the patient-led approach enabled participants to engage with therapy flexibly, in a timeframe that suited them. Because the approach is grounded in the principles of PCT, it acknowledges that people have different preferences and change will occur at different rates depending on the individual (Carey, 2011). The appropriate rate, number, and frequency of therapy sessions, therefore, can only be meaningfully determined by the patient (Carey et al., 2015).

To understand these data more, we asked participants about their experiences of receiving MOL using the patient-led appointment scheduling system (Griffiths, Mansell, Edge, Carey, et al., 2019). Importantly, participants were interviewed by a researcher who had not been involved in the delivery of the therapy and was blind to the therapeutic outcomes for the participants. Participants in this study were almost universally positive about the approach.

They valued the fact that sessions were available to them when needed. People described balancing therapy attendance with other demands on their time, such as work, childcare, and other healthcare appointments. One participant described the approach as providing a sense of safety because she knew that she could book appointments when she needed to, even during times when accessing therapy sessions was not a priority for her. Another participant talked about how being asked to attend sessions every week, irrespective of whether he thought that he needed to attend one, carried an implicit message that they were unwell or damaged in some way and, because of this, they should be attending therapy. The patient-led approach, in contrast, did not carry these negative connotations and was seen as more hopeful and empowering. The control that people experienced regarding how they booked therapy appointments mirrored the control they perceived themselves to have over what was discussed in MOL sessions. One participant described her experience of accessing MOL using patient-led scheduling in the following way:

> Yeah, so if a problem had come up, rather than getting upset and panicking about it, that I'm upset, 'How am I going to deal with this?' I'd think, 'Well, I don't have to wait longer than a week and I'll go and see [the therapist], and I'll be able to talk about it, and I'll deal with it'.
>
> (Griffiths, Mansell, Edge, Carey, et al., 2019, p. 7)

Current evidence base for Method of Levels in secondary care

In addition to a number of studies conducted in primary care (Carey et al., 2009; Carey & Mullan, 2008), as well as one carried out in a school setting (Churchman, Mansell, & Tai, 2019), several studies have investigated the use of MOL in secondary care settings. Carey et al. (2013) explored the use of MOL in a remote Australian secondary mental healthcare service. Part of this study involved the calculation of an 'efficiency ratio'. This is the ratio of effect size to mean number of sessions attended. When the efficiency ratio of this study was benchmarked against equivalent practice-based studies, the authors concluded that MOL was at least as effective, but significantly more efficient, than other psychological therapies. The study investigating the use of MOL and patient-led scheduling in early intervention in psychosis services, which was discussed earlier, found that the approach was feasible and acceptable to participants (Griffiths, Mansell, Carey, et al., 2019; Griffiths, Mansell, Edge, Carey, et al., 2019). Another study that explored the use of MOL in psychiatric inpatient settings found that the approach was acceptable and suitable for use in that context (Jenkins et al., 2020). Clearly, there is more research to be done in this area. We can now be reasonably confident, however, that it is possible to implement MOL in very diverse clinical areas. While adjustments to the infrastructure required to deliver therapy might be needed between settings, the principles underpinning MOL remain the same. There is also increasing evidence that patients find the approach helpful and acceptable (e.g., Griffiths, Mansell, Carey, et al., 2019; Griffiths, Mansell, Edge, Carey, et al., 2019).

Summary

For practitioners who are interested in increasing access to psychological interventions in secondary care, Method of Levels and patient-led scheduling represent exciting developments. They also signify a potential way forward for those of us who would like to see patients have more control over the kinds of professional help available to them and how they access support. Research conducted to date on MOL and patient-led scheduling has highlighted their potential to overcome some of the barriers that have traditionally prevented psychological interventions from becoming more widely available to users of secondary mental healthcare.

References

Beavan, V., Read, J., & Cartwright, C. (2011). The prevalence of voice-hearers in the general population: A literature review. *Journal of Mental Health*, *20*(3), 281–292. https://doi.org/10.3109/09638237.2011.562262

Beck, A. T., Steer, R. A., & Brown, G. K. (1996). *BDI-II, Beck depression inventory: Manual* (2nd ed.). Psychological Corp. Harcourt Brace.

British Psychological Society. (2009). *Code of Ethics and Conduct*. https://doi.org/10.2113/gsecongeo.52.2.198

Carey, T. A. (2005). Can patients specify treatment parameters? A preliminary investigation. *Clinical Psychology & Psychotherapy*, *12*, 326–335. https://doi.org/doi.org/10.1002/cpp.454

Carey, T. A. (2006). *The Method of Levels: How to do psychotherapy without getting in the way*. Living Control Systems Publishing.

Carey, T. A. (2008). Conflict, as the Achilles heel of perceptual control, offers a unifying approach to the formulation of psychological problems. *Counselling Psychology Review*, *23*(4), 5–16. http://psycnet.apa.org/record/2009-03454-003

Carey, T. A. (2009). Dancing with distress: Helping people transform psychological problems with the Method of Levels two-step. *The Cognitive Behaviour Therapist*, *2*(03), 167. https://doi.org/10.1017/S1754470X08000147

Carey, T. A. (2010). Will you follow while they lead? Introducing a patient-led approach to low intensity CBT interventions. In J. Bennet-Levy (Ed.), *Oxford guide to low intensity CBT interventions* (pp. 331–338). Oxford University Press. https://doi.org/10.1093/med:psych/9780199590117.003.0034

Carey, T. A. (2011). Exposure and reorganization: The what and how of effective psychotherapy. *Clinical Psychology Review*, *31*(2), 236–248. https://doi.org/10.1016/j.cpr.2010.04.004

Carey, T. A. (2016). Health is control. *Annals of Behavioural Science*, *2*(13), 1–3. http://behaviouralscience.imedpub.com/behavioural-science-psycology/health-is-control.pdf

Carey, T. A. (2017). *Patient-perspective care: A new paradigm for health systems and services* (1st ed.). Routledge.

Carey, T. A., Carey, M., Mullan, R. J., Spratt, C. G., & Spratt, M. B. (2009). Assessing the statistical and personal significance of the method of levels. *Behavioural and Cognitive Psychotherapy, 37*(3), 311–324. https://doi.org/10.1017/S1352465809005232

Carey, T. A., Kelly, R. E., Mansell, W., & Tai, S. J. (2012). What's therapeutic about the therapeutic relationship? A hypothesis for practice informed by Perceptual Control Theory. *The Cognitive Behaviour Therapist, 5*, 47–59. https://doi.org/10.1017/S1754470X12000037

Carey, T. A., Mansell, W., & Tai, S. J. (2015). *Principles-based counselling and psychotherapy*. Routledge. https://doi.org/10.4324/9781315695778

Carey, T. A., & Mullan, R. J. (2007). Patients taking the lead. A naturalistic investigation of a patient led approach to treatment in primary care. *Counselling Psychology Quarterly, 20*(1), 27–40. https://doi.org/10.1080/09515070701211304

Carey, T. A., & Mullan, R. J. (2008). Evaluating the method of levels. *Counselling Psychology Quarterly, 21*(October 2014), 247–256. https://doi.org/10.1080/09515070802396012

Carey, T. A., & Spratt, M. B. (2009). When is enough enough? Structuring the organization of treatment to maximize patient choice and control. *The Cognitive Behaviour Therapist, 2*(03), 211. https://doi.org/10.1017/S1754470X09000208

Carey, T. A., Tai, S. J., & Stiles, W. B. (2013). Effective and efficient: Using patient-led appointment scheduling in routine mental health practice in remote Australia. *Professional Psychology: Research & Practice, 44*(6), 405–414. https://doi.org/10.1037/a0035038

Churchman, A., Mansell, W., & Tai, S. (2019). A school-based feasibility study of method of levels: A novel form of client-led counselling. *Pastoral Care in Education, 37*(4), 331–346. https://doi.org/10.1080/02643944.2019.1642375

Fadden, G. (1997). Implementation of family interventions in routine clinical practice following staff training programs: A major cause for concern. *Journal of Mental Health, 6*(6), 599–612. https://doi.org/10.1080/09638239718464

Greenwood, K. E., Sweeney, A., Williams, S., Garety, P., Kuipers, E., Scott, J., & Peters, E. (2010). CHoice of Outcome In Cbt for psychosEs (CHOICE): The development of a new service user–led outcome measure of CBT for psychosis. *Schizophrenia Bulletin, 36*(1), 126–135. https://doi.org/10.1093/schbul/sbp117

Griffiths, R., Mansell, W., Carey, T. A., Edge, D., Emsley, R., & Tai, S. J. (2019a). Method of levels therapy for first-episode psychosis: The feasibility randomized controlled Next Level trial. *Journal of Clinical Psychology, 75*(10), 1756–1769. https://doi.org/10.1002/jclp.22820

Griffiths, R., Mansell, W., Edge, D., Carey, T. A., Peel, H., & Tai, S. J. (2019b). 'It was me answering my own questions': Experiences of method of levels therapy amongst people with first-episode psychosis. *International Journal of Mental Health Nursing, 28*(3), 1–14. https://doi.org/10.1111/inm.12576

Healthcare Quality Improvement Partnership. (2020). *How are secondary care psychological therapy services for adults with anxiety and depression performing?* www.hqip.org.uk/national-programmes

Ince, P., Haddock, G., & Tai, S. (2015). A systematic review of the implementation of recommended psychological interventions for schizophrenia: Rates, barriers, and improvement strategies. *Psychology and Psychotherapy: Theory, Research and Practice, 89*(3), 324–350. https://doi.org/10.1111/papt.12084

Jenkins, H., Reid, J., Williams, C., Tai, S., & Huddy, V. (2020). Feasibility and patient experiences of Method of Levels therapy in an acute mental health inpatient setting. *Issues in Mental Health Nursing*, 1–9. https://doi.org/10.1080/01612840.2019.1679928

Kay, S. R., Fiszbein, A., & Opler, L. A. (1987). The positive and negative syndrome scale (PANSS) for schizophrenia. *Schizophrenia Bulletin*, *13*(2), 261–276. www.ncbi.nlm.nih.gov/pubmed/3616518

Mansell, W., Carey, T. A., & Tai, S. (2013). *A transdiagnostic approach to CBT using method of levels therapy: Distinctive features*. Routledge.

Marken, R. S., & Carey, T. A. (2015a). *Controlling people: The paradoxical nature of being human*. Australian Academic Press.

Marken, R. S., & Carey, T. A. (2015b). Understanding the change process involved in solving psychological problems: A model-based approach to understanding how psychotherapy works. *Clinical Psychology and Psychotherapy*, *22*(6), 580–590. https://doi.org/10.1002/cpp.1919

Marken, R. S., & Powers, W. T. (1989). Random-walk chemotaxis: Trial and error as a control process. *Behavioral Neuroscience*, *103*(6), 1348–1355. https://doi.org/10.1037/0735-7044.103.6.1348

Miller, S. D., Duncan, B. L., Brown, J., Sparks, J. A., & Claud, D. A. (2003). The Outcome Rating Scale: A preliminary study of the reliability, validity, and feasibility of a brief visual analog measure. *Journal of Brief Therapy*, *2*(2), 91–100. https://pdfs.semanticscholar.org/a39c/ba5afb4f00fcd4af26df1937d9acaa448d21.pdf

National Institute for Health and Care Excellence (NICE). (2014). Psychosis and schizophrenia in adults: prevention and management. In *Nice*. https://doi.org/10.1002/14651858.CD010823.pub2.Copyright

Nursing and Midwifery Council. (2015). The Code: Professional standards of practice and behaviour for nurses, midwives and nursing associates. In *Midwives*. https://doi.org/10.1016/b978-075066123-2/50011-6

Powers, W. T. (1973). *Behavior: The control of perception*. Aldine.

Powers, W. T. (2005). *Behavior: The control of perception* (2nd ed.). Benchmark Publications.

Powers, W. T. (2008). *Living control systems III: The fact of control*. Benchmark Publications.

Powers, W. T., Clark, R. K., & Farland, R. L. M. (1960a). A general feedback theory of human behavior: Part I. *Perceptual and Motor Skills*, *11*(1), 71–88. https://doi.org/10.2466/pms.1960.11.1.71

Powers, W. T., Clark, R. K., & Farland, R. L. M. (1960b). A general feedback theory of human behavior: Part II. *Perceptual and Motor Skills*, *11*(1), 309–323. https://doi.org/10.2466/pms.1960.11.1.71

Royal College of Psychiatrists (2020). National Clinical Audit of Psychosis – National Report for the Early Intervention in Psychosis Audit 2019/2020. London: Healthcare Quality Improvement Partnership. www.rcpsych.ac.uk/NCAP

Runkel, P. J. (2003). *People as living things: The psychology of perceptual control*. Living Control Systems Publishing.

Spitzer, R. L., Kroenke, K., Williams, J. B. W., & Löwe, B. (2006). A brief measure for assessing generalized anxiety disorder: The GAD-7. *Archives of Internal Medicine*, *166*(10), 1092–1097. https://doi.org/10.1001/archinte.166.10.1092

Tarrier, N., Barrowclough, C., Haddock, G., & McGovern, J. (1999). The dissemination of innovative cognitive-behavioural psychosocial treatments for schizophrenia. *Journal of Mental Health*, *8*(6), 569–582. https://doi.org/10.1080/09638239917049

Valavanis, S., Thompson, C., & Murray, C. D. (2019). Positive aspects of voice-hearing: a qualitative metasynthesis. *Mental Health, Religion and Culture*, *22*(2), 208–225. https://doi.org/10.1080/13674676.2019.1601171

Varese, F., Tai, S. J., Pearson, L., & Mansell, W. (2016). Thematic associations between personal goals and clinical and non-clinical voices (auditory verbal hallucinations). *Psychosis*, *8*(1), 12–22. https://doi.org/10.1080/17522439.2015.1040442

Weiss, D. S., & Marmar, C. R. (1997). The impact of event scale-revised. In *Assessing Psychological Trauma and PTSD* (pp. 399–411). Guilford Press. https://psycnet.apa.org/record/1997-97162-013

Chapter 5

Adopting Perceptual Control Theory Principles in Mental Health Inpatient Settings and Other Restrictive Contexts

Introduction

A key concern of this book is the issue of maximising peoples' control over the support that they access from mental health services. The principles of Perceptual Control Theory (PCT; Powers, 1973, 2005a), which were introduced in Chapter 2, provide a theoretical basis for understanding why control is fundamental to health and wellbeing. As we have seen in Chapter 3, these principles can be used to inform the design of mental health services that adopt a 'patient perspective' approach to the delivery of care and have been tested in several studies (e.g., Carey et al., 2009, 2013; Griffiths, Mansell, Carey, et al., 2019). These principles also underpin the practice of Method of Levels (Carey, 2006), the psychological therapy described in Chapter 4 that aims to maximise patient control over the key parameters of therapy, such as choosing a problem focus, as well as factors such as the frequency and duration of therapy.

How do PCT principles apply, however, in contexts that are specifically designed to be restrictive? In situations, for example, where people are detained against their will, physically restrained, or given no choice about taking psychotropic medication. Although it is sometimes more subtle, care delivered outside of institutional settings can also be experienced as coercive and controlling. We will argue that PCT provides a coherent framework for understanding the practical and ethical challenges that can arise when working in restrictive environments. This chapter will consider working in environments that are restrictive by their design, such as locked inpatient wards, as well as staff practices that involve the use of restrictions, such as physical restraint. The overall aim of this chapter, therefore, is to consider how PCT principles can inform the approach taken by individual practitioners who are working in settings that impose some restrictions on the freedoms of patients. We will also consider how these principles can inform the design and underlying philosophy of services that could be experienced as restrictive. Primarily, we are referring to inpatient settings, but we will also discuss community mental healthcare practices that could be considered restrictive.

DOI: 10.4324/9781003041344-5

Background on restrictive practices: outline of policy and initiatives

In the 18th century and earlier, people with mental health difficulties residing in hospital facilities had to endure conditions described as 'inhumane', with patients 'locked in foul and unclean rooms with little light and/or held in manacles' (Newton-Howes, 2013, p. 422). The use of physical restraint and other deprivations of liberty continue to the present day. While staff routinely receive training in the safe implementation of these practices, there continue to be fatalities in inpatient mental health settings (Kersting et al., 2019), and patients often describe exposure to restrictive practices, such as physical restraint, as distressing (e.g., Cusack et al., 2018). In 2013, the United Kingdom charity MIND published a review of restrictive practices, which began with the following testimony:

> It was horrific … I had some bad experiences of being restrained face down with my face pushed into a pillow. I can't begin to describe how scary it was, not being able to signal, communicate, breathe, or speak. Anything you do to try to communicate, they put more pressure on you. The more you try to signal, the worse it is.
>
> (Mind, 2013, p. 2)

The Royal College of Psychiatrists have described the purpose of acute inpatient mental health services as being:

> to provide treatment when a person's illness cannot be managed in the community, and where the situation is so severe that specialist care is required in a safe and therapeutic space. Admissions should be purposeful, integrated with other services, as open and transparent as possible and as local and as short as possible.
>
> (Crisp et al., 2016, p. 16)

This setting provides a multidisciplinary approach to care with mental health nursing, occupational therapy, psychiatry, pharmacology, clinical psychology, and social work all providing input. During the past few decades, a process of deinstitutionalisation has taken place where care has increasingly been moved to community settings, rather than long-stay inpatient care. Consequently, there has been a steady decrease in the number of beds available for the purpose of inpatient mental health care (Garcia et al., 2005). This shift in policy was brought about partly by reports of abuse and neglect occurring in long stay hospitals and in an effort to reduce compulsory treatment (Cromby et al., 2013). However, mental health in-patient services in England and Wales have been highly criticised for overcrowding, lack of therapeutic activities, high staff turnover, and as being impoverished environments (Joint Commissioning Panel for Mental Health, 2013; Mind, 2013). Pressures on inpatient mental health services have been accompanied by efforts to shorten the length of hospital stays (Craig, 2016), which, in 2015, was an average of 32 days (NHS Benchmarking Network, 2019).

Despite the move towards deinstitutionalisation, there has been a gradual introduction of legislative powers that mean mental health services can exert more control over patients' lives in community settings. The introduction of the Community Treatment Order (CTO) in the UK is one such example (Department of Health, 2008). Series (2022) has referred to this blurring of lines between mental healthcare delivered in institutional and community settings as the 'invisible asylum'.

The legal framework regulating the use of restraint in the UK is the Mental Health Act (1983). This states that 'Physical restraint, rapid tranquillisation, seclusion and observation should only be used where de-escalation has proved insufficient and never as punishment.' Another relevant piece of UK legislation, The Mental Capacity Act (2005) states that the 'treatment and care provided to someone who lacks capacity should be the least restrictive of their basic rights and freedoms'. What is 'least restrictive' is not defined by the legislation, however. Instead, judgements of this kind might be guided by policy but are ultimately left to the discretion of the practitioner at hand. This situation is made even more problematic by the lack of evidence-based approaches that practitioners can draw on when they are seeking to implement alternatives to restrictive practices (Griffiths et al., 2021; Nawaz et al., 2021).

Restrictive practices and related concepts: definitions

There are several definitions of restrictive practice that are instructive for considering the main dimensions of the construct and its implications for patient care.

> Restrictive interventions are deliberate acts on the part of other person(s) that restrict a patient's movement, liberty and/or freedom to act independently in order to: take immediate control of a dangerous situation where there is a real possibility of harm to the person or others if no action is undertaken, and end or reduce significantly the danger to the patient or others. Restrictive interventions should not be used to punish or for the sole intention of inflicting pain, suffering or humiliation.
>
> (Department of Health, 2014, p. 14)

> Physical restraint is defined as any action or procedure that prevents a person's free body movement to a position of choice and/or normal access to his/her body by the use of any method, attached or adjacent to a person's body that he/she cannot control or remove easily.
>
> (Bleijlevens et al., 2016, p. 1)

The UK National Health Service defines restrictive practices as an activity that makes:

> someone do something they don't want to do or stopping someone doing something they want to do.
>
> (Skills for Care and Skills for Health, 2014, p. 9)

The purpose of restrictive practices is to reduce the risk a person's actions have to themselves or other people. In all of the examples provided above, the notion of inducing someone to do something they do not wish to do is mentioned. Thus, restrictive practices are about not only preventing actions but also inducing people to engage in actions they otherwise would not take. This is suggestive of coercion, which the Oxford English Dictionary defines as 'the application of force to control the action of a voluntary agent' (Oxford University Press, n.d., para 1). In the next section, we will examine the concept of coercion in the context of mental health treatment further.

Coercive practices and 'treatment pressures'

Szmukler and Appelbaum (2008) refer to interventions used to induce reluctant patients to engage in interventions as 'treatment pressures'. They describe a hierarchy of pressures that are presumed to represent a spectrum from low levels of clinician influence to interventions that represent high levels of influence. The lowest level can be illustrated with the example of a patient who is reluctant to take medication being informed by a practitioner about the possible unwanted effects of discontinuing medication. While the possibility of encountering unwanted effects might be a real concern, if the goal of the practitioner is to subtly encourage the patient to continue taking their medication, rather than to have a genuine conversation about the possible risks and benefits of taking medication, this could be considered coercive. At the highest level are compulsory interventions. An example of pressure at this level might include situations whereby discharge from hospital will only be facilitated if a patient takes medication. In the middle of the spectrum are approaches that rely on interpersonal leverage (e.g., the clinician expressing disappointment), inducements (e.g., tickets to sporting events), or threats to withhold benefits.

The highest levels of clinician influence in the hierarchy refer to 'formal' coercive practices. In many countries, including the United Kingdom, these practices are covered by legislation. Examples of clinician influence at this level would include the deprivation of liberty, detention, restricted freedom of movement, and enforced psychotropic medication. The lower-level examples described above, however, are often not covered by legal frameworks and are termed informal coercive practices, which can be contrasted with formal practices that require assent by statutory mechanisms. Informal coercive practices examined in recent qualitative research (Bendell et al., 2022; Pelto-Piri et al.,

2019; Rugkåsa et al., 2014) have reconsidered the examples given in the Szmukler and Appelbaum (2008) position paper. The use of inducements, for example, could reflect blackmail, trickery, or cheating. The phenomenon of informal coercion can be broadened to include a disciplinary style that, in one example, involved 'not saving any food if the patient was late for dinner' (Pelto-Piri et al., 2019, p. 3).

The range of the coercion spectrum can also be considered from the perspective of whether the interventions benefit or deprive the recipient of something they value. One end of the spectrum entails the clinician making an offer where the patient is free to consider some information or to receive a benefit in the form of extra assistance. The other end entails a threat where the patient may anticipate being 'worse off' by experiencing the deprivation of some right or obligation. Szmukler and Appelbaum (2008) note that what a clinician may perceive as an offer may be perceived as a threat by a patient. To illustrate this point, consider the following example. Imagine that an inpatient team are seeking the agreement of a patient to discharge them to a homeless hostel. To the team this is seen as an offer of accommodation that is a clear improvement on the ward conditions – it offers more autonomy. If, however, the patient does not want to be discharged to the homeless hostel – perhaps because they feel unsafe there – this offer would be seen as a threat. In this situation negotiation on the discharge plan would be needed for it to appeal to the patient – perhaps by offering discharge to bed and breakfast accommodation. If staff now make discharge to this accommodation conditional on taking medication, then the patient is likely to once again experience this as a threat. These nuances highlight the importance of the patient perspective in distinguishing what is coercive and what is collaborative care.

In contrast, the same patient may have discussed travelling to an end of season football game with their case worker. The case worker could make attending the football match contingent on the patient's consent to the discharge plan of moving to the homeless hostel. From the patient's perspective, the withdrawal of the offer to attend the football match may be greatly distressing and a profound threat. Where a specific coercive practice sits on the hierarchy described by Szmukler and Appelbaum (2008), therefore, appears to depend on the perspectives of the people concerned. In this example, what seems to be of lowest importance to the clinician is perceived to be of the highest importance by the patient, and vice versa.

Defining coercion

The preceding example highlights the perspective of the person being coerced. A systematic review of the literature on coercive practices in psychiatric settings identified a series of harmful themes such as feeling dehumanised or unheard by professionals (Newton-Howes & Mullen, 2011). Szmukler and Appelbaum (2008) note that:

> the subjective experience of being coerced may not follow what has been termed 'objective coercion'; that is, there is little correlation between patients' perceptions of being coerced and the actual use of, for example, civil commitment.
>
> (Szmukler & Appelbaum, 2008, p. 237)

The subjectivity of coercion is alluded to in the definition of coercion in the OED definition given earlier. The description of people being 'unwilling' indicates that the perspective of the person concerned is key to what is considered coercive because it is their will that is being transgressed. Newton-Howes and Mullen (2011) have introduced the concept of 'perceived coercion' to distinguish 'objective, external acts and internal, subjective attitudes' (p. 465). They state that coercion is 'best thought of as an internal subjective state, commonly referred to as "perceived coercion"' (Newton-Howes & Mullen, 2011, p. 465).

From an external to an internal perspective on coercion

In contrast to the definition of perceived coercion, some theoretical traditions attempt to consider coercion from an external perspective. For example, coercion theory (Patterson, 1982) offers a behaviourist perspective on the phenomenon, which was developed with the aim of understanding interpersonal dynamics within families. It understands the behaviour of individuals within a family as having a 'stimulus that elicits it and the consequences that maintain it. Events are conceptualised as either strengthening or weakening the stimulus response (S-R) bond' (Patterson, 1982, p. 85). The theory suggests that there are cycles of interaction between children and their caregivers that reflect the function of the behaviour of each. A child may react to a parent's request by refusing to comply, which in turn evokes anger in the parent, initially, but eventually the parent 'gives in'. This is believed to be reinforcing for both parties because the parent experiences some relief from the conflict, and the child does not have to comply with the initial request. The leading developer and populariser of behaviourism, B. F. Skinner, argued that attempts to control the behaviour of other people are likely to be experienced aversively by both the person being controlled and the person doing the controlling. According to Skinner, because

> of the aversive consequences of being controlled, the individual who undertakes to control other people is likely to be counter-controlled by all of them … the opposition to control is likely to be directed to the most objectionable forms – the use of force and conspicuous instances of exploitation [or] undue influence.
>
> (Skinner, 1953, p. 321)

The term counter-control, however, can be considered in the light of the more fundamental concept of control, which is defined from a PCT perspective in Chapter 2. One PCT-informed definition by Carey and Bourbon (2004) describes counter-control as an 'action taken by a controlee to systematically produce behavioural effects in a controller' (p. 4). The use of separate identifying terms – controlee and controller – might seem to imply that the controller and controlee are different in some way. This is not the case, however, if both people are understood as closed loop control systems, where each is in the environment of the other. This is an interaction between two people as the linking of two control systems through their shared environment (Bourbon, 1995). This notion is central to the understanding of how restrictive practices become problematic in a range of settings that is described in the remainder of this chapter. The shift from an external to an internal perspective on control is crucial to this endeavour.

An illustration of how an interaction between two people can work is depicted in Figure 5.1. This depicts two controlled perceptions, two references defining what state must be maintained, and two people able to act to stabilise their perceptions at the reference value. A key point is that the actions of each person do not just change their own perceptions. Because A and B are sharing the same environment, their actions also change the perceptions experienced by the other person.

Figure 5.1 illustrates how the environmental linkages are organised so that actions of each person 'disturb' the perceptions of the other. In many situations, these disturbances are easily countered so that the perception is quickly restored to the reference value and the disturbances do not have bothersome or problematic effects on the controlled variable. Indeed, the participant may not even notice the other person's presence or actions. An example of this is when

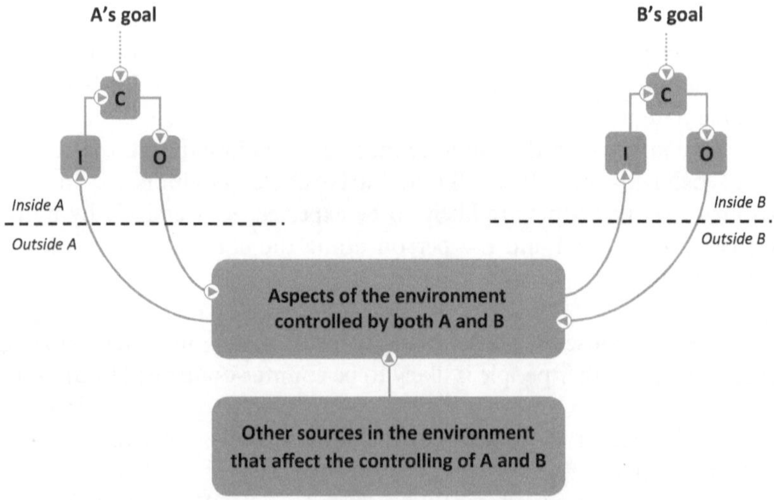

Figure 5.1 Interactions between closed negative feedback loops.

two people walk alongside each other across an open parkland. Person A might inadvertently drift closer to Person B than the latter would prefer. To correct this perception of proximity, Person B moves slightly away to allow more space. Given space is plentiful in the open area of the parkland, this could be done effortlessly. However, if this situation was to take place when the same people were walking along a narrow pavement alongside a busy road, it may be that Person B has no space to move and begins to experience discomfort because their preferred distance from Person A cannot be maintained. Figure 5.1 also highlights another way in which an environment may be configured so that output – for example, muscular movements, speech, or writing – have no effect on the perceptual variables Person A wishes to control. This is where the effects of Person B have greater force than those of Person A. For example, when held in a prone restrained position people cannot counter the stronger actions of the healthcare team. In this situation, the healthcare team represent an insuperable disturbance that renders the patient's attempts to control their perceptions ineffective. Even when the patient is straining with maximum muscular effort, the clinical team's actions have greater power than theirs, so the patient cannot move to their preferred position.

The origins of power imbalances

A definition of power is 'Capacity to direct or influence the behaviour of others' (Oxford University Press, n.d., para 2). By this definition the relationship between clinician and patient appears to be characterised by a power imbalance: the majority of the time, clinicians have greater capacity to direct the course of clinician–patient encounters than do patients. The example of prone restraint described above is one manifestation of this imbalance; the combined muscle forces of the team are greater than that of the individual patient. What is seldom acknowledged, however, is that holding the patient in such a position also has a consequence for the clinicians, who are also held in a static, albeit more comfortable, position. A crucial difference is that if one member of the restraining team wishes for a break, they are free to call a colleague to relieve them. This option is not available to the patient, so they have less capacity to control the situation. This unequal capacity to control events is an illustration of the power imbalance that exists between clinician and patient.

Figure 5.1 depicts how the patient's actions disturb the perceptions of the clinician and, if these perceptions are under control or deviate from the preferred state, the clinician must act to correct them. As just noted, however, the clinician may have several options to maintain control of the perceptual variable and, therefore, multiple alternative feedback paths from their actions to their perceptions that can be utilized to achieve their goal. The possibilities for the patient to meet their goal of being freed, however, are severely limited. Other than straining with all their might or trying to negotiate with the clinical team to free them, they have few other options to meet their goal. Thus, while clinician and patient inhabit the same environment there is an asymmetry in terms of their capacity to control their perceptions of that environment. Put another way, the clinician is afforded more degrees of freedom because they have more potential feedback paths at their disposal. Degrees of freedom in this instance refers to the variables describing a system that are free to change (Powers, 2005b). The location of an object in space has three degrees of freedom, X, Y, and Z. The location of an object on a flat surface has two degrees of freedom, X and Y. The location of an object attached to a rail running in the Y direction would have one degree of freedom left, X. Power imbalances are not just about the strength or any other characteristic of the clinician but how the environment they inhabit has been designed. It is both the healthcare system and the individual characteristics of clinicians that generate power imbalances.

In Reflection 5.1, Stuart describes a disagreement with staff that he had during his time as an inpatient of a mental health ward, and how the power held by staff impaired his ability to control things that he considered important.

Reflection 5.1 Stuart's experiences of inpatient mental health settings

The experience I'm going to talk about might sound trivial. But, to me, it's a good example of the kind of situation that can leave patients feeling like they have no control when they are in inpatient settings.

With the medication I'm prescribed, it's important to eat something before you take it. You don't want to take it on an empty stomach. During one inpatient stay, I asked if I could have some toast before I took my medication. The nursing assistant told me that they would not serve toast after 10:00 p.m., and, because it was 10:05 p.m., I would have to wait until the morning.

I felt frustrated that I didn't have any control over such simple things, like when I could eat a piece of toast. This resulted in an argument with the nursing assistant. They set off their personal alarm, and a group of burly men arrived and told me to settle down. This made me feel even more threatened. There was an implicit threat that if I did not do as I was told, this would result in me being restrained by the staff.

The reason given to me by the staff to explain why I could not have any toast was that they could not bend the rules and treat anyone differently. If they did, the whole ward system wouldn't work properly. So, they have to treat everyone exactly the same, otherwise it is unfair. But we're not all the same. Everyone doesn't have the same needs, and it doesn't make sense to design a system where that is not recognised.

The whole incident made me feel like I didn't have any control – even over something as basic as when to eat some toast – and I think it's a good example of how mundane disagreements can escalate into something more serious.

The origins of coercion

The example we described above, where a patient is being restrained by a clinical team, is a situation where an individual is unable to counter the actions of another group of people to correct the effects of this disturbance on a perception they are attempting to control. The stronger person (or group of people) forces the weaker to experience a particular state. In contrast, coercion refers to a situation where a coercee (the person experiencing the coercion) has to act in ways determined by the coercer to achieve and maintain a perceptual state the coercee does not wish to occur. As already made clear, PCT conceives of all behaviour as being purposeful, so 'acting against one's will' is not possible. There is a question of how this apparent contradiction comes about and this requires a further principle of PCT to be introduced, which is the principle of intrapersonal conflict. This is the conflict that arises within an individual and is described in Chapter 2. Figure 5.1 depicts two people pursuing one goal each. However, life necessarily involves the achievement of a multitude of goals. PCT conceives of a hierarchy of goals, with more abstract and global aspects of living at the top, such as a perception of oneself as a good parent, and more concrete strivings, such as taking one's daughter to music lessons, situated lower down the hierarchy. Thus, being a good parent is achieved by setting a goal of taking one's child to music lessons. The purpose of helping one's child attend the lessons, however, is to be a good parent.

The notion that it is possible to act 'against one's will' is addressed in PCT by the proposal that intrapersonal goal conflict can occur. A patient may be allowed to go home on leave for the weekend to see their elderly parent who is unable to travel to the hospital, for example, but only on the condition that they agree to take antipsychotic medication by intramuscular depot injection. This might create a conflict between goals relating to taking and not taking medication. The patient may wish to take their medication to achieve the goal of seeing their parent to be a good son or daughter. Being a good son or daughter, however, may also entail feeling energetic and conversational, something that could be impeded by taking medication. So, their experience of being a good son or daughter is impeded by the care team's stipulation of taking medication. While the patient might unwillingly accept the prescribed medication in order to pursue their goal of meeting with their parents, this approach will impair their ability to meet other goals, which could only be achieved by not taking medication.

Staff experiences of ethical dilemmas and inner conflict

The above example describes a conflict that may be experienced by a patient who has been informed that they must agree to accept an injection in order for them to be allowed leave to see their family. As noted by Hem et al. (2018), clinical management entailing this and similar scenarios involves ethical challenges, where a clinician may not have a clear idea of how best to proceed. This occurs when 'different values are at stake and oppose each other' (Hem et al., 2018, p. 93). The systematic review carried out by Hem et al. (2018) found that healthcare professionals felt a need to balance 'the therapeutic ideals of cooperation with the patient and their controlling role ... to create a safe and structured environment' (Hem et al., 2018, p. 100). In the context of the interacting loops described above, activities such as cooperating with a patient and maintaining a safe environment are both control processes. One reason that a clinician might feel a sense of discomfort is that neither of these goals is being satisfactorily achieved. Staff members are aware that, sometimes, their pursuit of a goal to ensure safety can cause patients' distress. A recent qualitative study on staff views on restrictive practices, for example, included the statement that they are 'a necessary evil' (Wilson et al., 2017, p. 500).

Conflict is undesirable not only because of the internal turmoil and emotional discomfort it generates for staff, but also because it undermines effective controlling (Powers, 1973). Where two control systems are controlling the same perceptual variable with maximum exertion but in opposing directions, the variable in question is easily influenced by disturbances. Imagine a tug of war taking place between two teams who are exactly matched in terms of strength and technique. At the point where the two teams are at maximum exertion, a small amount of influence by a third party in one direction or the other has the potential to tip the balance of the match in favour of one team. Although this example relates to a conflict between groups of people, the same principles apply in relation to intrapersonal conflicts. In a clinical setting, one manifestation of such a conflict might be staff appearing to act in an inconsistent or unpredictable manner.

Implications of this approach to understanding restrictive practices

The fundamental fact of unique, separate perspectives on decisions or choices is central to a PCT understanding of human interactions. This may appear self-evident but is worth saying because elsewhere notions of shared decision making are common. For example, there is a Shared Decision-Making Summary Guide published by the UK National Health Service (NHS England and NHS Improvement, 2019).

In the example described above, a patient may see contact with their parent as of paramount importance. Their clinical team, however, may take the view that completing the course of medication is the highest priority. Carey (2016) argues that the patient experience is paramount and should be the foundation of effective treatment. This has been formalised into a paradigm that places the patient's perspective as the key definer of treatment goals and resources (Carey, 2017).

As noted above, a coercer is themselves attempting to experience their own preferred states. One reason restraint of people in mental health settings is seen to be justified is that it contributes to the safety of other people. Newton-Howes and Mullen (2011) note that coercion might be a 'side effect of the actions taken by the health care professionals' (p. 465). If so, perceived coercion or abuse can be an unintended consequence of clinicians who are focusing solely on the narrow pursuit of a small number of goals. From their perspective, they wish to see the patient safe from harm or to prevent harm to others. Restrictive practices can be justified as being in the 'best interests' of the patient based on legal frameworks, such as the UK Mental Capacity Act (2005). The 'best interests' are informed by records of a person's past preferences, values, or those of family or others who can provide insight into these to substitute for the patient. Significant others are appointed by court officials or others deemed to be 'most engaged' in the person's care. This is problematic because a knowledge of a person's preferences could be limited, inaccurate, or used coercively, as in the example relating to taking medication that is given above. By focusing on the expected perspectives of the patient, the authentic perspective of the patient could be neglected. The only person capable of offering a truly authentic perspective on an individual's preferences, is the person themselves. There are indications, however, that personal preferences are not prioritised sufficiently. For example, a recent review into the provision of inpatient care in the UK positioned the patient's perspective fourth in a list of priorities for assessments, behind their symptoms, risks, and family history (Crisp et al., 2016).

Reflection 5.2 describes Stuart's experience of being detained in hospital and unable to engage in an activity that he valued – in this case, smoking. His

Reflection 5.2 Stuart's reflections on being detained in a restrictive environment

Although I'm aware of the negative impact this has on my physical health, I'm still a smoker.

This became a real problem for me when I was admitted to a mental health inpatient unit. There was only one smoking area on the ward, and this was locked off all day apart from at three designated smoke breaks. This was the case, even though I would estimate that 70% of the patients on the ward were smokers.

When it was time for a smoke break, a nurse or nursing assistant would escort everyone to the smoking area, light everyone's cigarettes, and observe us while we smoked. We were then brought back onto the ward.

Having a cigarette became a real point of contention between patients and staff. For many patients, having a cigarette was seen as an integral part of their day. Staff, however, saw smoke breaks as a chore that could be dropped if other tasks came along that were seen as more important. 'If we're busy, we can't do it', seemed to be their attitude.

Some patients would try and use their Section 17 leave [A section of the UK's Mental Health Act (1983) that enables detained patients to have short periods of leave from the ward] to go for a cigarette. Nursing staff would try to stop this because they said this was not a therapeutic activity. It makes me wonder who gets to decide whether an activity is therapeutic or not.

Limiting access to the smoking area seemed like a paternalistic, top-down decision from the managers. They have decided that they are a non-smoking Trust, and that's the end of it. This approach doesn't take patients' views into account.

When you don't have control over the big things in your life (e.g., leaving the ward or the medication you are taking), losing control over the smaller things, like smoking, leaves you all at sea. It makes you feel like you are in a constant state of flux, unable to make good decisions about your care. This approach doesn't recognise the minutiae of life that becomes very important when your liberty is taken away.

Situations like this also seem to make the ward environment more chaotic. It creates conflict between nurses and patients, and these little disputes build up over the course of a day. Eventually, the general feeling of dissatisfaction leads onto bigger problems on the ward, such as incidents of violence and aggression.

Even worse, the antagonism created by situations like this is often pathologized. It is viewed as a symptom of a mental health problem, rather than as an understandable reaction to the limitations of the ward environment.

I think giving patients more control over things that they prioritise could help avoid a lot of the problems that we see on mental health wards.

reflections on this experience highlight the damaging consequences of limiting people's ability to control things that they consider to be important and failing to take into account the preferences of patients.

Patient and staff perspectives

We next attempt to illustrate staff and patient perspectives by including contributions from people with experience of inpatient mental health services. The first perspective was provided by a nurse with experience of working inpatient mental health settings. One of this book's authors (Jasmine) also responded, drawing on her experience of inpatient care. To obtain these perspectives we presented

Vignette 5.1 Conflict in a ward environment

Chris is a 23-year-old man who is currently an inpatient on an acute mental health ward. He is detained under Section 3 of the Mental Health Act. Over the last few days, Chris has described hearing voices that tell him to harm himself and to end his life. He reports feeling frightened by the voices but says that he is able to resist their commands. Chris usually lives with his parents and is very keen to leave the ward and return home. He says that he does not find medication helpful and, consequently, does not want to take the antipsychotic medication that has been prescribed for him. When Chris attends his weekly ward round, which is also attended by his father and members of the multidisciplinary team, he says that he wants to be discharged from hospital. Chris' father says that he supports his son's view that leaving hospital would be the best option, but he wants Chris to start taking his medication before he is discharged. On hearing this, Chris becomes frustrated and begins to shout aggressively at both his father and the ward's clinical staff. He quickly leaves the meeting room where the ward round is taking place, shouting that he is 'getting out of here, no matter what!'

the contributors with a vignette, which, although fictional, was designed to be a realistic scenario reflecting the crises and tensions that occur in this environment. We chose to use a vignette to elicit the perceptions and goals of the two contributors in a situation they would both be familiar with but whose goals could be distinct.

The contributors' responses are below, with interviewer prompts included in bold font. As mentioned, the patient perspective is provided by one of the books authors (Jasmine) who has experience of inpatient care. The staff perspective to the hypothetical scenario is provided by a mental health nurse with experience of working in inpatient environments.

What would you do next?

Staff perspective: 'Go to speak to him and verbally deescalate. Find out what's going on and what is frustrating him. Try to work out a plan to try and mediate between him and the ward round or the doctors. Try to get him back into the ward round'.

Patient perspective: 'When someone is really aggressive or violent, everybody will kind of look the other way. [I would] wait for them to be calmer and then check in with them going "did it not go well are you feeling really squished, like a caged Tiger?" I'd definitely go to them and be like, "calm down, bring it down, you've got leave scheduled for next week when you're going to see your family – you don't want to lose that now"'.

Why would it be important for you to do this next?

Staff perspective: 'Initially, trying to deescalate is part of maintaining the hospital environment. Safety is our main priority and making sure other people are safe. Initially what you have to do before you can do anything else is to try and calm him down. Then you can look at his treatment, which is, again, our priority. Work with him so he can help with his treatment plan because he's going to be the one doing it. If he's not happy, he's not going to comply, and the doctors are not going to let him out of hospital if he's not working with his treatment plan, which he needs to be co-designing with the doctors and his family. Getting him involved is how it works because if people aren't involved within their treatment plan, then often the treatment plan doesn't work. His aggression and frustration will only get worse if he's ignored within the treatment plan'.

Patient perspective: 'Firstly, selfish reason – [for me] to feel calm and tranquil. Second, wanting other people who are more vulnerable or quiet or less vocal with their body language to feel at peace. Finally, to make sure that Chris is ok, to make sure he feels listened to. Considering he's come from that environment where he's clearly really frustrated and angry … to kind of [be a] middle ground for him and be, like, "Ok, you don't want to take the medication but actually smashing up the ward isn't going to make it any better"'.

The staff member was asked a follow-up question on a possible conflict between goals of safety and helping people get well, and stated, 'it comes down to is the person aggressive and frustrated because they are in hospital, and are they are being given medication that they don't want, or it is because they are unwell. [This] is quite difficult to see sometimes – people might be unwell, but it can be massively heightened by being in an inpatient setting. Risks might be reduced massively by being at home and not being in that environment. Trying to … work with Chris and try to meet him halfway, almost, in what he believes is going to be good for him'.

Synthesis

Both the staff and the patients stated that it would be important to speak to Chris about how the ward round went. They both also mention the importance of a safe environment. In the case of the patient perspective, this relates to experiencing a sense of tranquillity, to allow other people to be at peace. The staff perspective introduces the importance of the treatment plan with the added notion that this can only be successful if Chris is involved in this. The staff perspective also describes the possible importance of treatment, specifically medication.

This exercise highlights that, whilst staff and patients might be in the ward environment for very different reasons, their preferences for the state of this environment might be similar and perhaps in surprising ways. Indeed, some aspects of what might be assumed to be solely the goals of staff members, such as talking to and supporting patients, might be taken on by other patients. This is consistent with the importance of informal help in this setting (Galloway & Pistrang, 2019). However, as we have been discussing through this volume, some of these goals – taking medication, for example – might not be viewed as helpful from Chris's perspective. Nonetheless, if ward staff, managers, and policymakers become more aware of the goals of patients and staff, it might be possible to create environments that are less likely to cause conflict and loss of control.

Key messages for staff and commissioners

Services should focus on helping patients achieve their preferred perceptual states and, where possible, try to avoid mandating their behaviour. The current approach to working with patients in inpatient settings is to reduce the frequency of behaviours seen to pose a risk to the self and others. An obvious example of this might be self-harm behaviour. Self-harm is understood to both pose a risk to the self – by injury – but is also acknowledged to serve a function, which might be to be an external expression of pain, a distraction technique, or an attempt to punish oneself (Mind, 2022). From a PCT perspective these are two sides of the same coin, the self-harm behaviour is fulfilling the purpose to maintain the inner perceptual state. Crucially, the behaviour side of the loop might be achieved through many different means, but the reference value or goal must be held static. Therefore, services that attempt to change behaviour, without considering its purpose will not be effective and might be harmful. The focus of help should be on restoring individual's control over inner states and not mandating behaviour change.

Practitioners working in restrictive settings should maintain a stance of curiosity and creativity. To a certain extent, this point overlaps with the points made in the preceding section, but is of central importance, so warrants specific attention. As we have been making clear throughout this volume, we suggest that psychological change requires four key ingredients to be present – external expression of a problem, sustained focus on that problem, accompanying emotion during this process, and, finally, a shift in perspective. Ward environments severely restrict the first of these – patients often report they are unable to talk freely about their difficulties (Staniszewska et al., 2019). The environment is also prescriptive about what treatment entails and what change should entail – this hinders rather than helps the recovery process. Furthermore, attempts to control the behaviour of patients act as a disturbance to the patient's controlling. The consequence of this is that patients often put their energy into counteracting staff's efforts to control their behaviour, rather than focusing on the elements of recovery described above. For this reason, a clearer focus on setting up conditions where people can talk freely about their reasons for admission – and what problems they are facing in their life – would allow the change process to happen.

The stance of curiosity towards a problem creates an opportunity to broaden and deepen a person's awareness of the problem itself. Most importantly, the aim of increasing awareness needs to apply to the whole system, not just the user of the services. Often, it is the practitioners who have the greater capacity to shift their goals such that coercion, restriction, or force are not evident; the judgement of risk versus benefit and the power to make a decision on this basis lie within the staff rather than the patient, and so staff also need space and a sense of authentic curiosity to explore their competing goals.

Within a situation of coercion, curiosity can provide the space for all to consider their choices in the light of the multiple goals they hold, most of which will be held outside of awareness during day-to-day life. For example, as an example of coercion, a clinician may choose not to share detailed information about the potential side effects of medication with a patient. They may do this with only one goal in mind, such as, 'to make sure the patient takes their medication to stay well'. There may be no conscious deliberation of how the patient might stay well through other means, such as forming honest and open relationships with health professionals, and even less consideration of whether coercing a patient to take medication could make their problems worse. Within supervision, a colleague may ask themselves, 'What are the advantages of not telling the patient about the side effects?' or 'What might be the issues with not sharing this information?' This would raise the clinician's awareness of other important goals that they hold in these situations – to practice in a transparent and honest way, for example. The process of reflecting on a multitude of relevant goals might help to limit the use of coercive measures, such as the one described in this example.

From the perspective of the patient, we have pointed out that instances of coercion require the existence of goal conflict. So, for example, the patient in the above example may also want to keep taking the medication as the main means to stay well, and so, not considering the potential side effects of the medication and not considering various other means to stay well may provide the straightforward kind of help that he wants, in addition to minimising disagreement with a health professional. Yet, it would be curious questioning that might reveal this, and in turn provide the potential for a new perspective to emerge, such as, 'Maybe it is more important for me to explore other ways of keeping well than it is for me to convince myself that there is a simple solution and to "keep the peace" with my prescriber'. Of course, although there is no guarantee that such awareness-raising exercises will necessarily lead to a beneficial outcome for all parties, it will lead to all parties being better informed. Such an approach also increases the likelihood that staff–patient interactions are more honest and respectful of each person's autonomy.

A key question is how to time the process of 'awareness raising' within a busy service. Should all clinical decisions be questioned by an independent party before they are made? Can reflective questioning after the event help to resolve the continued distress experienced and help to revise the staff practice going forward? These questions may need to be answered in practice but, given that they reflect the timescales with regard to the experience of restrictive practices, this may serve as a guide: retrospective questioning is helpful for forming a better understanding of a restrictive interaction and for preparing for similar situations in the future. The use of a brief conversation with an independent, curious listener (such as a trained professional or user representative who doesn't know the patient) before and after the use of restrictive practices is one approach that services could trial. Careful practice-based data collection could clarify the benefits and costs of the approach.

The foregoing recommendations make clear that space to talk and reflect is essential for services to negotiate and ensure safe practice. This entails the provision of resources – most obviously increased staffing – to allow these discussions to take place. PCT positions resources on the environment side of the loop. They may protect the perceptual variable under control from disturbances or act as part of a feedback function. The notion of degrees of freedom is also helpful for understanding how patients and staff can regain control of perceptions that are important to them. Ward environments need to be designed so that there are sufficient degrees of freedom for patients and staff to meet their respective goals. Degrees of freedom can be created by the provision of resources that enrich the environment; these might include greater outside space, a variety of recreational activities, private space when requested, and so on. Whilst providing patients with a wide variety of activities and choice in the sensory qualities of the ward can clearly be helpful, however, it is not possible to know what all patients and staff preferences might be. For this reason, an optimal environment would allow residents to make changes to the spaces they inhabit during an episode of care. In essence, we are arguing for a responsive environment where patients can control key parameters of the environment to increase their capacity to maintain control over important perceptual variables. The ward might not be the same place when a patient has left it, it could grow organically and become enriched over time. This is notable when patients share artwork or pottery to enrich the environment for others. As Powers (2005b, p. 233) stated 'Our goal structures must be such that there are many actions that would serve to satisfy any given goal; the richer the store of alternatives the more likely we are to minimise conflict and maintain control'.

This highlights the key point that environments that excessively restrict degrees of freedom foment conflict and loss of control.

Designing ward environments

The provision of resources in the ward environment must be designed and considered carefully. How ward environments are designed is discussed in UK clinical guidelines for the management of violence and aggression in inpatient wards (National Institute for Health and Care Excellence (NICE), 2015). They advise that ward environments should unlock doors where possible, include enhanced decoration, use a simplified layout, and provide access to outside spaces. The purpose of inpatient mental health care goes beyond simply managing aggressive behaviour – the primary purpose is, arguably, the alleviation of distress and to provide a nurturing environment that facilitates reorganisation, enabling intrapsychic conflicts to be resolved. A relatively recent systematic review found scarce research focused on ward design (Papoulias et al., 2014), and the limited evidence available highlighted the importance of privacy to patients admitted to inpatient wards. From a PCT perspective, the preservation of privacy was presumably deemed so important by patients because it enabled them to maintain important perceptual states within acceptable parameters and minimised disruptions that would otherwise impair the effective control of these states.

As already noted, what may be a fundamental principle of ward design, from a PCT perspective, is the importance of allowing sufficient degrees of freedom for control over desired perceptual states. Furthermore, having control might entail choosing not to partake in the resources that are offered, or choosing not to engage with others. Also, using such an approach, staff merely offer resources, and avoid advising or suggesting that certain activities might be helpful for people. As Carey (2017, p. 59) notes, health professionals should 'minimise the extent to which they teach, coach and guide and maximise the time they spend enquiring, offering and following'. This means that resources are available for patients who are not pushed or cajoled into using them.

The preceding discussion does not, however, address the important question of how the resources are chosen in the first place. The obvious place to start is the patient perspective and for this purpose Jasmine Waldorf has suggested a series of possible resources that might be provided in a ward environment that would have been useful and therapeutic from her perspective. These are summarised in Table 5.1.

It is important to note that, while the aspects of a therapeutic environment identified by Jasmine in Table 5.1 might share some similarities with the preferences of other people admitted to inpatient wards, there are also likely to be significant differences between peoples' views about what they consider to be an optimal ward environment.

Table 5.1 Jasmine's perspective on therapeutic aspects of ward environments and how these features relate to lower- and higher-level goals

Aspect of the ward environment	*Lower-level goals*	*Higher-level-goals*
A quiet space to connect with the staff on duty and discuss feelings, emotions, and life events.	– To talk to staff and have perspectives heard – Have a natural conversation	– Regain a sense of self – Being connected and social – Egalitarian culture
A loud space with loud TV or music playing at a high volume	– Cope with voices, anger, frustration, or painful feelings	– Express feelings
Solitary space in your private room to comfort eat and sleep and rest.	– Quiet time – Time away from others	– Space for health and reflection – Independence
A creative space with art materials or an activity like colouring, drawing, or self care (nail art club etc.)	– Express ideas nonverbally – Pass time constructively	– Creative lifestyle
Outside space with plants and vegetable patch, where wild birds or insects can visit	– Relax – Feel connected to nature – Sense of freedom	– An outdoors lifestyle – Sustaining nature

Summary

We began this chapter by describing the widespread adoption of restrictive practices in acute and secondary care mental health services. There is little evidence that the autonomy of patients and their ability give voice to their perspective has increased in recent decades. Lasting and meaningful change to these conditions requires a coherent understanding of how services should be organised to achieve safer, more efficient, and more effective care. We have described how PCT could achieve such an understanding. Coercion or force, for example, are understood by PCT as manifestations of either insufficient space for awareness to fully explore – and fully inform – decision making or arising from limitations in the available degrees of freedom that environments provide for patients and staff to achieve control. If services focus on these principles – rather than mandating the behaviour of patients or staff – this will allow for the restoration of control of perceptual states and, ultimately, a widespread perception that inpatient services are moving towards being places of safety, healing, and recovery.

References

Bendell, C., Williams, C., & Huddy, V. (2022). Exploring experiences of restrictive practices within inpatient mental healthcare from the perspectives of patients and staff. *Journal of Psychiatric Intensive Care*, *18*(1), 17–29. https://doi.org/10.20299/jpi.2022.005

Bleijlevens, M. H. C., Wagner, L. M., Capezuti, E., & Hamers, J. P. H. (2016). Physical Restraints: Consensus of a Research Definition Using a Modified Delphi Technique. *Journal of the American Geriatrics Society*, *64*(11), 2307–2310. https://doi.org/10.1111/jgs.14435

Bourbon, W. T. (1995). Perceptual control theory. In H. L. Roitblat & J. Meyer (Eds.), *Comparative Approaches to Cognitive Science* (pp. 151–172). MIT Press.

Carey, T. A. (2006). *The Method of Levels: How to do psychotherapy without getting in the way*. Living Control Systems Publishing.

Carey, T. A. (2016). Health is control. *Annals of Behavioural Science*, *2*(13), 1–3. http://behaviouralscience.imedpub.com/behavioural-science-psycology/health-is-control.pdf

Carey, T. A. (2017). *Patient-perspective care: A new paradigm for health systems and services* (1st ed.). Routledge.

Carey, T. A., & Bourbon, W. T. (2004). Countercontrol: A new look at some old problems. *Intervention in School and Clinic*, *40*(1), 3–9. https://doi.org/10.1177/10534512040400010101

Carey, T. A., Carey, M., Mullan, R. J., Spratt, C. G., & Spratt, M. B. (2009). Assessing the statistical and personal significance of the method of levels. *Behavioural and Cognitive Psychotherapy*, *37*(3), 311–324. https://doi.org/10.1017/S1352465809005232

Carey, T. A., Tai, S. J., & Stiles, W. B. (2013). Effective and efficient: Using patient-led appointment scheduling in routine mental health practice in remote Australia. *Professional Psychology: Research & Practice*, *44*(6), 405–414. https://doi.org/10.1037/a0035038

Craig, T. K. J. (2016). Shorter hospitalizations at the expense of quality? Experiences of inpatient psychiatry in the post-institutional era. *World Psychiatry*, *15*(2), 91–92. https://doi.org/10.1002/wps.20320

Crisp, N., Smith, G., & Nicholson, K. (2016). Old problems, new solutions – improving acute psychiatric care for adults in England. *The Commission on Acute Adult Psychiatric Care, February*, 1–6. www.rcpsych.ac.uk/pdf/Old_Problems_New_Solutions_CAAPC_Report_England.pdf

Cromby, J., Harper, D., & Reavey, P. (2013). *Psychology, mental health and distress* (pp. xxix, 420). Palgrave Macmillan/Springer Nature. https://doi.org/10.1007/978-1-137-29589-7

Cusack, P., Cusack, F. P., McAndrew, S., McKeown, M., & Duxbury, J. (2018). An integrative review exploring the physical and psychological harm inherent in using restraint in mental health inpatient settings. *International Journal of Mental Health Nursing*, *27*(3), 1162–1176. https://doi.org/10.1111/inm.12432

Department of Health. (2008). *Mental Health Act 2007: Patients on after-care under supervision (ACUS): transitional arrangements*.

Department of Health. (2014). *Positive and proactive care: Reducing the need for restrictive interventions*. https://assets.publishing.service.gov.uk/government/uploads/system/uploads/attachment_data/file/300293/JRA_DoH_Guidance_on_RP_web_accessible.pdf

Mental Capacity Act, (2005).

Galloway, A., & Pistrang, N. (2019). 'We're stronger if we work together': experiences of naturally occurring peer support in an inpatient setting. *Journal of Mental Health (Abingdon, England)*, *28*(4), 419–426. https://doi.org/10.1080/09638237.2018.1521925

Garcia, I., Kennett, C., Quraishi, M., & Durcan, G. (2005). A measure of concerns. *Mental Health Today (Brighton, England)*, 29–31.

Griffiths, R., Dawber, A., McDougall, T., Midgley, S., & Baker, J. (2021). Non-restrictive interventions to reduce self-harm amongst children in mental health inpatient settings: Systematic review and narrative synthesis. *International Journal of Mental Health Nursing*, 1–16. https://doi.org/10.1111/inm.12940

Griffiths, R., Mansell, W., Carey, T. A., Edge, D., Emsley, R., & Tai, S. J. (2019). Method of levels therapy for first-episode psychosis: The feasibility randomized controlled Next Level trial. *Journal of Clinical Psychology*, *75*(10), 1756–1769. https://doi.org/10.1002/jclp.22820

Hem, M. H., Gjerberg, E., Husum, T. L., & Pedersen, R. (2018). Ethical challenges when using coercion in mental healthcare: A systematic literature review. *Nursing Ethics*, *25*(1), 92–110. https://doi.org/10.1177/0969733016629770

Joint Commissioning Panel for Mental Health. (2013). *Guidance for commissioners of acute care: Inpatient and crisis home treatment*. 25. http://www.jcpmh.info/wp-content/uploads/jcpmh-acutecare-guide.pdf

Kersting, X. A. K., Hirsch, S., & Steinert, T. (2019). Physical harm and death in the context of coercive measures in psychiatric patients: A systematic review. *Frontiers in Psychiatry*, *10*, 400. https://doi.org/10.3389/fpsyt.2019.00400

Mental Health Act, (1983). https://doi.org/10.1201/9781315380797

Mind. (2013). *Physical restraint in mental health crisis care: A briefing for MP*. www.mind.org.uk/media-a/4373/for-mps.pdf

Mind. (2022). *Self-harm*. www.mind.org.uk/information-support/types-of-mental-health-problems/self-harm/about-self-harm/

National Institute for Health and Care Excellence (NICE). (2015). Violence and aggression: short-term management in mental health, health and community settings. *Nice, May 2015*, 1–64.

Nawaz, R. F., Reen, G., Bloodworth, N., Maughan, D., & Vincent, C. (2021). Interventions to reduce self-harm on in-patient wards: Systematic review. *BJPsych Open*, *7*(3), 1–9. https://doi.org/10.1192/bjo.2021.41

Newton-Howes, G. (2013). Use of seclusion for managing behavioural disturbance in patients. *Advances in Psychiatric Treatment*, *19*(6), 422–428. https://doi.org/10.1192/apt.bp.112.011114

Newton-Howes, G., & Mullen, R. (2011). Coercion in psychiatric care: Systematic review of correlates and themes. *Psychiatric Services (Washington, D.C.)*, *62*(5), 465–470. https://doi.org/10.1176/ps.62.5.pss6205_0465

NHS Benchmarking Network. (2019). *2019 Mental Health (Inpatient/CMHT) project – Results published*. www.nhsbenchmarking.nhs.uk/news/2019-mental-health-inpatientcmht-project-results-published

NHS England and NHS Improvement. (2019). *Personalised Care Shared Decision Making Summary guide NHS England and NHS Improvement*. 1–14.

Oxford English Dictionary. (n.d.). Oxford University Press.

Papoulias, C., Csipke, E., Rose, D., McKellar, S., & Wykes, T. (2014). The psychiatric ward as a therapeutic space: Systematic review. *British Journal of Psychiatry*, *205*(3), 171–176. https://doi.org/10.1192/bjp.bp.114.144873

Patterson, G. R. (1982). *Coercive family process* (Vol. 3). Castalia publishing company.

Pelto-Piri, V., Kjellin, L., Hylén, U., Valenti, E., & Priebe, S. (2019). Different forms of informal coercion in psychiatry: A qualitative study. *BMC Research Notes*, *12*(1), 787. https://doi.org/10.1186/s13104-019-4823-x

Powers, W. T. (1973). *Behavior: The control of perception*. Aldine.

Powers, W. T. (2005a). *Behavior: The control of perception* (2nd ed.). Benchmark Publications.

Powers, W. T. (2005b). Degrees of freedom in social interactions. In *Living control systems: Selected papers of William T. Powers* (2nd ed., pp. 221–236). Benchmark Publications.

Rugkåsa, J., Dawson, J., & Burns, T. (2014). CTOs: What is the state of the evidence? *Social Psychiatry and Psychiatric Epidemiology*, *49*(12), 1861–1871. https://doi.org/10.1007/s00127-014-0839-7

Series, L. (2022). Introduction. In *Deprivation of liberty in the shadows of the institution* (1st ed., pp. 1–11). Bristol University Press. https://doi.org/10.2307/j.ctv2fjwpsp.8

Skills for Care and Skills for Health. (2014). *A positive and proactive workforce*. www.skillsforcare.org.uk/Documents/Topics/Restrictive-practices/A-positive-and-proactive-workforce.pdf

Skinner, B. F. (1953). *Science and human behavior*. Sage. https://doi.org/10.4135/9781483327372.n6

Staniszewska, S., Mockford, C., Chadburn, G., Fenton, S. J., Bhui, K., Larkin, M., Newton, E., Crepaz-Keay, D., Griffiths, F., & Weich, S. (2019). Experiences of in-patient mental health services: Systematic review. *British Journal of Psychiatry*, *214*(6), 329–338. https://doi.org/10.1192/bjp.2019.22

Szmukler, G., & Appelbaum, P. S. (2008). Treatment pressures, leverage, coercion, and compulsion in mental health care. *Journal of Mental Health*, *17*(3), 233–244. https://doi.org/10.1080/09638230802052203

Wilson, C., Rouse, L., Rae, S., & Kar Ray, M. (2017). Is restraint a 'necessary evil' in mental health care? Mental health inpatients' and staff members' experience of physical restraint. *International Journal of Mental Health Nursing*, *26*(5), 500–512. https://doi.org/10.1111/inm.12382

Chapter 6

Towards a Perceptual Control Theory-Informed Framework for Ethical Decision Making in Secondary Mental Healthcare

Introduction

In this book, we have argued that adopting Perceptual Control Theory (PCT) principles might contribute to the development of secondary care mental health services that, in addition to being more effective and efficient, are more humane. From a PCT perspective, central to the idea of behaving 'humanely' is treating people according to their preferences for how they want to be treated. There are clearly occasions when due to medical reasons people are unable to express their preferences (e.g., in cases of coma or brain injury). Yet practitioners working in secondary mental healthcare are also sometimes required to engage in activities that explicitly contradict people's expressed preferences. Examples of such activities include detaining people against their will, using physical restraint and seclusion, and enforcing medication. Practitioners, therefore, are frequently required to balance conflicting ethical principles in their clinical decision making. Where someone is deemed to be at an immediate risk of harming themselves, for example, at what point is it ethical to limit that person's ability to act autonomously with the aim of preventing future harm? Much has been written on the topic of ethics and mental health, and the purpose of this chapter is not to provide an exhaustive overview of the area. Instead, we have two aims. First, to consider how PCT might provide a novel and useful perspective for understanding ethical constructs commonly discussed in the mental health literature. Second, to provide a practical PCT-informed framework that might help practitioners to resolve ethical dilemmas that they encounter in their practice.

Perceptual Control Theory and ethics

The Oxford English Dictionary defines ethics as 'The branch of knowledge or study dealing with moral principles' and 'A system or set of moral principles' (Oxford University Press, n.d., para 1). PCT, on the other hand, is a theory of behaviour that provides an explanation of how preferred states are maintained and achieved through hierarchical negative feedback control. PCT does not

DOI: 10.4324/9781003041344-6

contain within it an intrinsic code of ethics. Nor does it offer prescriptive instructions to help us distinguish between the morality of actions that might be considered right or wrong. To illustrate this point with an analogy, understanding the physics of how to convert vast amounts of nuclear potential energy into kinetic energy tells you nothing about whether it is ever ethical to deploy nuclear weapons during international conflicts. That said, definitions of ethics, or moral philosophy as it is otherwise known, make it clear that this is a branch of philosophy that is primarily concerned with what humans do and how they behave. White (2017) offers the following description of ethics:

> The simplest way to describe what ethics does is to say that it *evaluates human actions*. It's a particular way of making *positive and negative judgments* about what we ourselves and other people do.
>
> (White, 2017, p. 2)

Nuttall's (1993) description also describes ethics as being concerned with the morality of our actions:

> Morality is concerned with right and wrong, good and bad, virtue and vice; with judging what we do and the consequences of what we do. Moral philosophy, or ethics, is that branch of philosophy which has morality as its subject matter.
>
> (Nuttall, 1993, p. 1)

Ethics, therefore, is concerned with what humans *do*. Consequently, a robust understanding of the phenomenon of human behaviour seems essential. From our perspective, ethical decision making is likely to be enhanced when we possess a coherent understanding of what behaviour is and is not. In this chapter, we will present the argument that PCT is generally consistent with existing ethical frameworks that are commonly used by practitioners. Further, we will argue that understanding behaviour from a PCT perspective deepens our understanding of *why* the principles contained within these approaches to ethics are so important to the practice of mental healthcare.

It is often assumed that ethics sits outside scientific enquiry, and it is this apparent objectivity that allows ethical reviews, advice, and decision making with regard to scientific research and its clinical applications. Yet, the science of ethics is a long-established field, dating back at least as far as Leslie Stephen's seminal volume that explained ethics through the lens of evolution via natural selection, intrinsic and extrinsic motivation, emotional reasoning, free-will, and consciousness (Stephens, 1882). Clearly, psychology is a field of enquiry that can inform an understanding of motives, intentions, and capacity for decision-making, and there is a contemporary basis for the psychology of ethics based upon this empirical work (Mallon & Doris, 2013). Rather than review this literature, the focus of this chapter will be to pinpoint how PCT provides a unique perspective on the science of ethics.

One unique feature of PCT is the precision with which PCT specifies a small number of principles of how living things, including humans, function. This, in turn, leads to only a small number of recommendations for practice that apply universally, rather than an array of guidelines and policies for various contexts, individuals, and ethically challenging situations. Those principles are control, conflict, and reorganisation. So, in a nutshell, ethical decisions, just like any other decision, involve the balanced exploration of conflicting goals within, across, and between individuals, such that a higher-level perspective is accessed, often spontaneously through reorganisation, from which a relatively better informed, and more inclusive, set of decisions can be made. These 'decisions' would be located at successively lower levels in the hierarchy and might include policies (at a principle level), procedures (at a program level), or responsibilities (at a relationship level), for example.

Yet, PCT is not designed to inform decision making for specific ethical dilemmas. Rather, it is a framework that reminds all of us that some degree of error and conflict is an inevitable feature of any complex system, and therefore monitoring, feedback, and seeking out mistakes, complaints, exceptions, and discrepancies is necessary for its smooth functioning; and that a perspective that encompasses all parts of that system is likely to be more adaptive. In essence therefore, a PCT informed view on ethics proposes that, like in Method of Levels therapy, problems should be sought out and explored rather than avoided, and that a curious stance to help broaden awareness could be used to help address any ethical dilemma so that a solution can be found that is considered helpful from the perspective of the person dealing with it.

Framework for biomedical ethics

Within a context where many approaches to ethics have been proposed, we focus on the approach that is specifically developed for the biomedical domain and is the most widely accepted and used. This is a framework by Beauchamp and Childress (2019). They have proposed a framework for biomedical ethics that consists of four principles: respect for autonomy, beneficence, non-maleficence, and justice. The approach is now the most widely taught framework for understanding biomedical ethics for people training as healthcare professionals, and it is commonly used by practitioners to inform their ethical decision making (Page, 2012). In this section, we will explore each of these four principles in turn and consider how they might be understood in the context of PCT.

Respect for autonomy

The principle of respect for autonomy asserts that people should be free to make choices based on their personal goals and values. It is not sufficient for others to merely not interfere with autonomous decision making. Where necessary and appropriate, people should be given the support they need to pursue personally meaningful goals. Beauchamp and Childress (2019) acknowledge that there are limits to the principle of respect for autonomy. Circumstances can arise where it might be justifiable to override someone's preferences in order to comply with competing ethical principles – in situations where someone's actions might cause others harm, for example. They also argue that competence (the ability to perform a task) could be considered a necessary precondition for autonomy, although they acknowledge that 'competence' and 'incompetence' are not binary conditions. These states exist on a continuum that is specific to the task being performed. Respecting the principle of respect for autonomy is fundamental to adopting a PCT perspective to mental healthcare. According to PCT, humans can be said to be in a state of health when they are able to control perceptions of important psychological, social, and biological variables in line with internally generated goals specifying the state of those variables (Carey, 2016). Where people are unable to control perceptual variables according to their goals, this can be distressing, harmful, and even life threatening. Respecting autonomy can be considered ethical, therefore, because adopting this principle maximises opportunities for people to work towards personally meaningful goals; to create the life that they want for themselves. It is for this reason that clinical applications of PCT, such as the patient-led appointment scheduling system described in Chapters 3 and 4, endeavour to increase patients' control over how they can engage with healthcare resources.

Nonmaleficence

The principle of nonmaleficence, according to Beauchamp and Childress's (2019) framework, means that there is an obligation not to inflict harm on others. Enacting this principle, of course, requires a working definition of what is meant by the term 'harm'. Beauchamp and Childress (2019) argue that, in this context, harm refers to impeding or thwarting someone's interests. From a PCT perspective, not respecting the principle of nonmaleficence could be understood as situations where someone is needlessly prevented from controlling important perceptual variables in line with their preferences for the state of those variables. Consider a situation, for example, where a patient discloses distressing past experiences to a health professional, and their preference is for that information to remain within their immediate care team. Should the health professional subsequently share these details with other individuals or organisations, this could be considered harmful because it impedes the patient's ability to meet their goal of limiting others' access to this information. Of course, there might be situations where it is ethical to override the preferences of the patient and share this information, such as in cases where sharing the information could potentially limit or prevent harm to third parties.

Beneficence

Distinct from the principle of nonmaleficence, which relates to the avoidance of actions that cause others harm, the principle of beneficence stipulates that healthcare professionals have a duty to promote and protect the interests of the people they are working with (Beauchamp & Childress, 2019). While this might initially sound relatively straight forward, and is consistent with the expectations of many professional guidelines (e.g., the Nursing and Midwifery Council's (NMC) Code of Conduct for registered nurses (Nursing and Midwifery Council, 2015), or the Health and Care Professionals Council's (HCPC) standards for conduct (HCPC, 2016) in the UK), ethical decision making becomes more complicated in situations where there is conflict between the principles of autonomy and beneficence, such as where a patient declines support or treatment that the practitioner strongly believes will be helpful. This can lead to the impulse in practitioners to override the autonomy of patients and adopt a more paternalistic approach to treatment. These dilemmas can arise in all areas of healthcare but seem particularly problematic in the field of mental health, where views on topics such as how psychological distress should be conceptualised and what constitutes an effective treatment are deeply contested. Where there is a large degree of uncertainty about the outcomes of a particular treatment and lack of clarity about the mechanisms through which that outcome will be achieved, as often appears to be the case in the field of mental health, the ethical justification for overriding a patient's autonomy becomes more questionable.

Beneficent actions, from a PCT perspective, are those that increase the patient's capacity to control perceptual variables that they consider important, enabling them to reduce intrinsic error. Whether or not a particular action is truly beneficent, therefore, can only be judged from the perspective of the person the practitioner is seeking to help. This means that it is important for practitioners to keep an open mind about patients' goals, and to avoid making assumptions about what will or will not be considered helpful. Remaining curious about patients' goals, and actively enquiring about these, will increase the likelihood that practitioners' actions are experienced as beneficent.

If a patient is homeless, for example, and they are finding it difficult to meet their goal of accessing stable accommodation due to the complexity of the housing system, providing practical support to enable the patient to achieve this goal could be considered a beneficent action. In this situation, the actions of the healthcare professional have increased the patient's ability to reduce the difference between their goal (to secure stable housing) and their current perception of the state of that variable (no stable housing). In PCT terms, the practitioner in this situation could be considered part of the feedback function for the patient, because they are acting as a resource to enable them to reduce intrinsic error between their current and desired perceptions. One of this book's authors (Robert), however, has experience of working with patients who expressed a preference for *not* being housed in stable accommodation, and resisted efforts from health and social care workers to provide this for them. Despite the evidence of the deleterious effect that homelessness can have on physical and mental health (Onapa et al., 2022), in situations like this, it is less clear that actions such as arranging stable housing should be considered a beneficent act in all cases, particularly when those actions are inconsistent with the preferences of patients.

Justice

The fourth ethical principle identified by Beauchamp and Childress (2019) is that of justice. In this context, this principle largely pertains to distributive justice (how rights and responsibilities are distributed throughout a society), as opposed to criminal and other forms of justice. It concerns issues such as how finite healthcare resources can be shared equitably and fairly amongst members of a society. Beauchamp and Childress (2019) highlight that numerous theories have been proposed that seek to determine how rights, responsibilities, and resources can be distributed fairly. These include utilitarian theories (e.g., we should prioritise those actions that are of overall benefit to society), libertarian theories (e.g., issues relating to the distribution of resources are best left to market forces), and egalitarian theories (e.g., resources should be distributed equally amongst society). There has been a large body of research that focuses on addressing problems of health inequity (e.g., Marmot, 2015; Pickett & Wilkinson, 2015). Carey, Tai, and Griffiths (2021) have adopted a PCT perspective to argue that issues relating to health inequity are a side effect of problems such as a relatively small number of people focusing on the accrual of wealth, without giving due consideration to the effects this has on other people's ability to maintain control over important aspects of their lives. Inequities relating to access to healthcare and other vital resources arise, they argue, because the controlling of a powerful minority disrupts the controlling being carried out by other less powerful members of society. At a societal level, one implication of this perspective is that healthcare policy, and other related policies, should be designed to maximise the controlling of all members of society, not just a powerful minority. Exactly how this ambition can be achieved, however, is still a matter for debate.

The framework proposed by Beauchamp and Childress (2019) is, of course, just one of many to have been proposed. We have spent some time discussing the work of Beauchamp and Childress (2019), however, because this framework has proved particularly influential in the field of healthcare (Page, 2012).

PCT principles for ethical decision making

A PCT framework for ethical decision making would start with a recognition that we are all controllers. Different groups of people who are in contact with mental health services – including patient, practitioners, relatives, managers, healthcare commissioners, policy makers, researchers – are all seeking to control their perceptions in line with references specifying the preferred state of those perceptions. When human behaviour is viewed from this perspective, it is possible to propose a series of principles, informed by PCT, that might inform ethical decision making:

Respect other people's controlling

It is important to acknowledge and, where possible, respect people's controlling nature. It is not always possible to tell what variables someone is controlling merely by observing their behaviour (Willett et al., 2017), particularly when they are experiencing high levels of distress. Practitioners should endeavour, however, to understand the goals of the patients they are working with. This can be achieved by asking curious questions and carefully observing people's behaviour.

Avoid impeding people's controlling

Where possible, we should avoid acting in a manner that unnecessarily thwarts or impairs the controlling being carried out by other people. Once we have a good sense of the goals that are important to someone, aside from in exceptional circumstances, it is not ethical to seek to prevent them from reaching these goals. Practitioners should also be mindful of the fact that they may not fully understand what goals someone is seeking to control (Willett et al., 2017). In PCT terms, we should aim to avoid acting as an unnecessary disturbance to the controlling being performed by other people.

Act as a resource that enhances people's controlling

In addition to avoiding acting as a disturbance to people's controlling, practitioners should take active steps to support the controlling being carried out by patients. In essence, this means healthcare services and professionals should act as resources to enable patients to regain or maintain control over variables that they consider personally meaningful.

Address the conditions that disrupt effective controlling

The environmental conditions in which people live play a significant role in determining how effectively they can maintain control over important psychological, social, and biological variables. Overwhelming environmental forces (or 'insuperable disturbances') make it impossible for people to maintain control, irrespective of the amount of effort expended to achieve this. It is ethical, therefore, to endeavour to create conditions that support people's controlling.

This could be achieved by addressing interpersonal, societal, economic, and political factors that unnecessarily disrupt people's controlling.

These principles are broadly consistent with those found in existing ethical frameworks for healthcare, such as Beauchamp and Childress's (2019) principles of autonomy, nonmaleficence, beneficence, and justice. You might reasonably ask at this point, what is the unique contribution that PCT makes to this area if the ethical principles that follow from the theory are similar to those from existing frameworks? From our perspective, there is an advantage to having ethical principles that are grounded in an accurate understanding of the nature of living things. Of course, not everyone will be convinced that PCT has the potential to provide an accurate understanding of human behaviour, and more work is certainly required to test the fundamental tenets of the theory. That is why the title of this chapter rather tentatively suggests that we need to move *towards* a PCT-informed framework for ethical decision making. Our position is that *if* PCT does indeed provide the accurate model of behaviour that it purports to (and, as described in Chapter 1, for which there is already some good evidence), then the principles listed above could be used to inform ethical decision making in the field of mental healthcare.

Resolving ethical conflicts

Practitioners working in mental health will inevitably experience conflicts between ethical principles on a routine basis. Powers (2005) defined intrapersonal conflict as situations where a person is seeking to meet two incompatible goals at once. Faced with a situation where a patient is cutting themselves with a razor blade, for example, a mental health nurse working in a mental health inpatient ward might experience a conflict between wanting to respect the autonomy of the patient to make choices for themselves, while also wanting to physically intervene to minimise harm to the patient. In another example, a psychiatrist working in a community mental health team might feel reluctant to detain a patient under mental health legislation because they want to respect the person's right to continue to live independently, even when the person appears highly distressed. The psychiatrist, however, might also want to detain the patient to prevent the person's mental health from deteriorating further. Since the psychiatrist cannot meet their 'detain the patient' and 'do not detain the patient' goals simultaneously, they are in a state of conflict.

Morgan et al. (2015) have suggested that conflict over values – including conflict over ethical values – is the norm in the field of mental health. They argue that the way to work with this is to bring these conflicting values into awareness and to avoid supressing them. We would agree with this approach. As an aside, from a PCT perspective, the term 'value' is one of many possible synonyms that all refer to the same thing: a reference value. This is a reference specifying the state of a particular perceptual variable. Goals, wishes, preferences, desires, hopes, ambitions, are just a few of the other terms that people commonly use to describe reference values. Returning to the issue of conflict,

PCT proposes that a person's ability to control is disrupted when reference values at the same level within the perceptual hierarchy are in conflict. The way people resolve these kinds of intrapersonal conflicts is through a process called reorganisation. As described in Chapter 2, sustaining awareness on conflicting goals facilitates reorganisation. Powers (2009) proposed that it is this process of sustaining awareness on conflicts that is the effective component of all psychological therapies. In Chapter 4, we provided an overview of the Method of Levels (MOL), which is an approach to psychotherapy that directly applies PCT. Therapists using MOL aim to direct a person's awareness towards the source of conflicts, supporting the reorganisation process. It is possible, however, to apply the same principles that support effective MOL in contexts other than psychotherapy. Most of us have had the experience at some time of informally talking to a friend about a problem, when, seemingly out of the blue, a new perspective on the issue comes to mind. You might also have experienced 'Eureka!' or 'Aha' moments at some unexpected juncture. Maybe when you are driving, or listening to music, or taking a walk, or mowing the lawn. These are all examples of the reorganisation process at work.

Conflicts between ethical principles in the field of mental healthcare are likely to be specific to the individual and the context in which they occur. It is unlikely to be helpful, therefore, to provide prescriptive advice about how to resolve conflicts between specific ethical principles because this approach ignores these important individual and contextual factors. What PCT can offer, however, is a theoretically informed approach to creating the conditions necessary to enable key stakeholders (including patients, practitioners, relatives, and others) to resolve conflicts between competing ethical principles.

First, people in conflict need to be able to talk openly or find some other means of expressing whatever it is that is that is troubling them. One reason for this is that resolving conflicts is, essentially, a creative process. The reorganisation system is not finding a solution to the conflict that already exists somewhere within the perceptual hierarchy. This is not the mental equivalent of rifling through a filing cabinet to find a pre-existing solution that fits the bill (as would be the case with accessing a memory of solving a similar problem in the past). Instead, the reorganisation system is creating a bespoke solution to the problem; one that did not exist previously (for example, by prioritising exploration and discovery over safety). The process of reorganisation is supported when people are able to talk freely and without inhibitions about whatever is on their mind in that moment (Carey et al., 2015). The idea that free expression is associated with creativity is not a new one. The German playwriter Friedrich Schiller (1759–1805) for example, eloquently expressed a similar idea when he argued that creativity was enhanced when new ideas are not filtered or supressed:

> In the case of a creative mind, however, the intelligence has withdrawn its watchers from the gates, the ideas rush in pell-mell, and it is only then that the great heap is looked over and critically examined.
>
> (Letter of 1 December 1788, quoted in Freud (1913, p. 86))

Second, people's reorganising will be supported when they are able to shift and sustain their awareness onto the source of the conflict long enough for it to be resolved. In MOL sessions, this is achieved by the therapist paying attention for 'disruptions' (signs of momentary shifts in awareness onto potentially relevant background thoughts) and then asking about these.

For people who are experiencing conflicts between ethical principles, therefore, what is required is a context where they can talk freely about conflicts, accompanied by some means of being encouraged to pay attention to related background thoughts. The opportunities and resources available to enable this process will vary between stakeholders. Clinical supervision might be one context where practitioners can talk openly about conflicts between ethical principles. Informal peer support and multidisciplinary team meetings might also provide this opportunity. Interactions between patients, carers, and practitioners – such as ward rounds, community visits, or outpatient appointments – might also be settings where there are opportunities to support the reorganisation process. Differences in perceived power between these parties, however, might mean that it is not possible for everyone to talk openly about what is on their mind. We explore this issue in more depth later in this chapter.

Increasing the available degrees of freedom

Ethical decision making is complicated further when we consider the fact that someone's goals in the here-and-now might not be the same as the goals they might hold in the future. There is evidence, for example, that patients who have been detained under mental health legislation have ambivalent views on the experience, depending on when they are asked about this. In one report on the subject (Hemmington et al., 2021), people reported that the process of being detained was severely distressing at the time:

> I remember [...] being terrified [...] I think it was a complete sense of loss of control [...] something was happening to me and it was very scary.
>
> (Hemmington et al., 2021, p. 52)

Longer term, however, some people had a sense that being detained under mental health legislation was an appropriate course of action during periods of extreme distress:

> [Being sectioned] saved my life basically because I'm not in my right mind when I'm doing these sort of things [...] so, thankfully, the last time they didn't even give me the option to go voluntarily [...] looking back it was the right decision, even though I've hated being in hospital.
>
> (Hemmington et al., 2021, p. 49)

When practitioners are faced with a binary choice between using legislation to detain a patient whose life is considered to be at risk or taking no action, detaining the patient is likely to be viewed as the more ethical response, even where the patient objects to this. The ethics of designing a mental health system with a severely limited repertoire of available support for patients to access during periods of distress are more questionable.

Alternatives to mental health inpatient units have been developed that seek to avoid compulsory detention and have less focus on the use of psychotropic medications. One such approach is the model proposed by the Soteria Network, which focuses on creating drug-free or minimal-medication environments for people experiencing 'psychosis' and extreme distress (www.soterianetwork.org.uk/).

Other alternatives to psychiatric inpatient admissions include the use of resources such as 'crisis houses' and 'safe havens'. Expanding such options increases the 'degrees of freedom' available to patients who are seeking support. As discussed in Chapter 5, in this context, the term degrees of freedom refers to the number of available pathways that are open to someone who is striving to meet a specific goal (Powers, 1989). If someone is experiencing extreme levels of distress, and is actively seeking support for this, but the only option open to them is to be admitted to a mental health inpatient unit, then the degrees of freedom available to them are quite limited. One implication of this is that it is ethical to expand the range of options that are available to patients seeking support from mental health services to help them regain control. This increases the likelihood that people can access timely support that they consider to be relevant and helpful.

There is evidence that the limited range of options for supporting people in extreme distress also creates problems for practitioners. One qualitative study reported that mental health nurses perceived restraint and seclusion to be barbaric but felt like they had no choice but to use these practices because resource issues (e.g., sufficient staff, training, and education) meant that there was limited scope for using alternative approaches (Hawsawi et al., 2020). The authors conclude:

> These negative experiences of seclusion and restraint created an internal conflict between nurses' moral judgement of providing coercive free care and their professional duty in maintaining safety and managing violence.
>
> (Hawsawi et al., 2020, p. 842)

Increasing the degrees of freedom available to mental health staff with regard to the diversity of approaches they can offer patients, therefore, appears to be ethically justified.

Power differences

A key issue implicit in the earlier sections of this chapter is that a recognised power imbalance exists between users of mental health services and the professionals who work for them. It is, therefore, important to establish the meaning of 'power' within the context of PCT. Essentially, power is the capacity to exert control. In the context of two or more individuals, a power imbalance indicates that one person or group can more effectively exert control over something that also matters to another person or group. Clearly, within the realms of mental health services, this includes the capacity for professionals to offer or withhold treatment or other forms of help. Within inpatient services it can include the capacity to offer or withhold some more basic liberties, such as the freedom of movement, access to other people, and access to a range of commodities that would be available outside the hospital setting. Power imbalances can also make it easier for patients to be coerced into activities by professionals as a genuine or apparent part of their treatment, such as completion of therapy 'homework', taking certain medications, or following certain advice. At an extreme, power imbalances may make it easier for emotional, physical, or sexual abuse to occur. Issues around imbalances of power are, therefore, critical to understand and address.

Given the potential harmful effects of power imbalances, one might assume that it is best addressed by attempting to remove the power imbalance directly. As we work through the issues below, however, it will hopefully become evident that the most effective form of intervention is, again, likely to be ways to help raise people's awareness of their conflicts and higher-level goals. Classically, Method of Levels can provide this both for patients and professionals, if they wish to use it.

The principle focus of many psychological interventions is to help *empower* users of mental health services. Indeed, this has been the focus of many elements of this book, such as the shift towards patients booking their own appointments, choosing how much therapy they need, and choosing to talk about what they want to talk about in therapy. In this regard, empowering users also has an impact on *disempowering* professionals with regard to their control of these specific variables. Yet, it is clear from PCT that people control many aspects of their lives, and so giving control to patients will only disturb professionals if variables such as problem focus and therapy duration matter to them – that is, if these variables form some of the perceived aspects of important higher-level goals, such as 'to be an influence on my patients' or 'to be seen as knowledgeable'. PCT makes it clear that people are control systems – people counteract attempts by others to reduce control over what matters to them. Attempts to disempower powerful individuals who do not wish to relinquish control over the variables in question will be met with resistance. Therefore, professionals who are concerned about the implications of patient empowerment for themselves and their profession may benefit from talking to a colleague who listens carefully about these concerns and asks curious questions, as one would expect within MOL.

In the authors' experience, we have met considerable resistance to the idea of disempowerment by fellow mental health professionals. Yet, we have also engaged colleagues in some deeper exploration of their concerns and discovered that many can entertain disempowerment of certain elements of their services after discussion. Quite often, this emerges after exploring the wider benefits for patients that might emerge from their capacity to control certain elements of their treatment. It is a salutatory reminder that many of the 'recommendations' in this book are in themselves attempts to utilise the power imbalance implicit within the perceived superiority of academic knowledge of scientific theory and research in order to 'persuade' colleagues of the benefits of shifting the power imbalance between clinicians and patients. As such, any supervisor, manager, and policy maker reading this book needs to bear in mind their own position of power. This involves looking into ways that they can facilitate an even-handed and collaborative approach to the raising of awareness within their staff regarding these issues, rather than instigating changes without consultation. The struggle of an MOL therapist to remain impartial whilst continuing to ask curious, searching questions, is paralleled by the struggle of a service manager to remain impartial when engaging their clinical staff with the potential for systemic change that may shift the balance of power to the benefit of the patients' well-being and mental health.

In Reflection 6.1, Stuart gives his thoughts on how power imbalances can manifest themselves within mental health inpatient settings. It is clear that his perception of the unequal distribution of power within the inpatient setting impaired his ability to maintain effective control over factors that he considered important, such as his capacity to express himself openly. This is concerning, given the importance of all parties feeling able to express themselves openly, which we have attempted to emphasise throughout this book.

Summary

In this chapter we have argued that PCT principles are broadly consistent with current paradigms in biomedical ethics. Further, we have proposed that the perspective on human behaviour that PCT affords can be used to develop our understanding of the importance of key ethical principles. Conflicts between ethical principles in the field of mental healthcare are almost ubiquitous. PCT provides a framework that can be used to design healthcare systems and practices that support the resolution of intrapersonal and interpersonal conflicts relating to ethical principles that can occur within and between service users and providers. Crucially, the resolution of such conflicts requires a milieu where people are encouraged to reflect deeply on their own conflicting goals, to be curious about the goals of others, and to feel comfortable in expressing themselves openly. This will not only support people to resolve

Reflection 6.1 Stuart's experiences of power imbalances

My take is that there are power imbalances in every aspect of mental health services. This might be overt coercive behaviour, such as the threat of using physical restraint and forced intramuscular injection of medication, or it can be more subtle. I think there is an underlying message that says, 'If you don't do what we want you to do, we'll lock you up until you comply'.

One example of how these power imbalances can play out happened while I was an inpatient of a mental health ward. I was unhappy with a number of aspects of my care. I got to the point of completing a formal complaint form. I then pulled back from this and decided not to submit the form. I felt like any complaint made against staff could have negative connotations for my care. The staff have so much power over all aspects of your life. Where you sit for dinner, how quickly your food is served, whether your questions get answered, and how staff respond to your needs. Whatever you ask for, you can be put to the back of the queue.

This created a real conflict for me. I wanted to be able to express myself and speak up about my needs and the aspects of my care that I thought were poor. But I didn't want to alienate the staff and was worried about the possible repercussions of doing so.

There are so many influences on the behaviour of staff (e.g., their training and education, their goals as a practitioner, the ward culture, healthcare policy, and practice guidelines). Staff need to have an awareness of how much power they have and how they are exerting control over patients' lives. This is so built into the system at the moment that I don't think many staff are aware of how they are controlling patients and the impact this has on patients' wellbeing and right to agency. I think some staff get caught up in a 'key jangling' culture of locking doors and treating wards like they are prisons, whereas they are actually working in a hospital.

We need to find a way to create cultures in mental health settings that give patients more control over what they do and what they can say.

their own intrapersonal conflicts relating to ethical dilemmas, but, hopefully, it will also encourage practitioners to relinquish some control over those aspects of healthcare delivery that would be better placed in the hands of patients. Finally, increasing the overall degrees of freedom available to patients regarding the kinds of support they can access could reduce the reliance of the mental healthcare system on coercive and restrictive practices that are fraught with ethical difficulties.

References

Beauchamp, T. L., & Childress, J. F. (2019). *Principles of biomedical ethics* (8th ed.). Oxford University Press.

Carey, T. A. (2016). Health is control. *Annals of Behavioural Science*, *2*(13), 1–3. http://behaviouralscience.imedpub.com/behavioural-science-psycology/health-is-control.pdf

Carey, T. A., Mansell, W., & Tai, S. J. (2015). *Principles-based counselling and psychotherapy*. Routledge. https://doi.org/10.4324/9781315695778

Carey, T. A., Tai, S. J., & Griffiths, R. (2021). *Deconstructing health inequity: A perceptual control theory perspective*. Palgrave Macmillan.

Freud, S. (1913). *The interpretation of dreams*. MacMillan.

Hawsawi, T., Power, T., Zugai, J., & Jackson, D. (2020). Nurses' and consumers' shared experiences of seclusion and restraint: A qualitative literature review. *International Journal of Mental Health Nursing*, *29*(5), 831–845. https://doi.org/10.1111/inm.12716

HCPC. (2016). Standards of conduct, performance and ethics. *The Health and Care Professions Council*, 1–17. www.hcpc-uk.org/globalassets/resources/standards/standards-of-conduct-performance-and-ethics.pdf

Hemmington, J., Graham, M., Marshall, A., Brammer, A., Stone, K., & Vicary, S. (2021). Approved mental health professionals, best interests assessors and people with lived experience – An exploration of professional identities and practice. In *Mental Health* (Issue May). www.socialworkengland.org.uk/media/4046/amhp-bia-research-report.pdf

Mallon, R., & Doris, J. M. (2013). The science of ethics. In *The Blackwell Guide to Ethical Theory* (pp. 169–196). Blackwell. https://doi.org/10.1111/b.9780631201199.1999.00010.x

Marmot, M. (2015). *The health gap: The challenge of an unequal world* (1st ed.). Bloomsbury Publishing.

Morgan, A., Felton, A., Fulford, B., Kalathil, J., & Stacey, G. (2015). *Values and ethics in mental health: An exploration for practice* (1st ed.). Bloomsbury Publishing.

Nursing and Midwifery Council. (2015). The Code: Professional standards of practice and behaviour for nurses, midwives and nursing associates. In *Midwives*. https://doi.org/10.1016/b978-075066123-2/50011-6

Nuttall, J. (1993). *Moral questions: An introduction to ethics* (1st ed.). Polity.

Onapa, H., Sharpley, C. F., Bitsika, V., McMillan, M. E., MacLure, K., Smith, L., & Agnew, L. L. (2022). The physical and mental health effects of housing homeless people: A systematic review. *Health and Social Care in the Community*, *30*(2), 448–468. https://doi.org/10.1111/hsc.13486

Oxford English Dictionary. (n.d.). Oxford University Press.

Page, K. (2012). The four principles: Can they be measured and do they predict ethical decision making? *BMC Medical Ethics*, *13*(1), 10. https://doi.org/10.1186/1472-6939-13-10

Pickett, K. E., & Wilkinson, R. G. (2015). Income inequality and health: A causal review. *Social Science & Medicine (1982)*, *128*, 316–326. https://doi.org/10.1016/j.socscimed.2014.12.031

Powers, W. T. (1989). *Living control systems: Selected papers of William T. Powers*. Control Systems Group.

Powers, W. T. (2005). *Behavior: The control of perception* (2nd ed.). Benchmark Publications.

Powers, W. T. (2009). PCT and MOL: A brief history of Perceptual Control Theory and the Method of Levels. *The Cognitive Behaviour Therapist*, *2*(3), 118–122. https://doi.org/10.1017/S1754470X08000111

Stephens, L. (1882). *The science of ethics*. Cambridge University Press.

White, T. I. (2017). *Right and wrong: A practical introduction to ethics* (2nd ed.). Wiley-Blackwell.

Willett, A. B. S., Marken, R. S., Parker, M. G., & Mansell, W. (2017). Control blindness: Why people can make incorrect inferences about the intentions of others. *Attention, Perception, and Psychophysics*, *79*(3), 841–849. https://doi.org/10.3758/s13414-016-1268-3

Chapter 7

Working with Relatives and Carers of People Using Secondary Mental Healthcare

Introduction

In this chapter, we explore the contribution that Perceptual Control Theory (PCT; Powers, 2005; Powers, 1973) might make to addressing problems that can occur within the close personal relationships of people accessing secondary mental healthcare. Finding effective ways to resolve such difficulties could lead to improved outcomes for both relatives and patients. Although more general cybernetic approaches to family therapy have been proposed (e.g., Keeney & Ross, 1983), to our knowledge, no research has yet been conducted that directly applies PCT to the field of family interventions in secondary mental healthcare. Our hope is that this chapter highlights some potential opportunities for developing effective, PCT-informed approaches to working with families, and that this will provide the impetus for future research in this area. After discussing research relating to the experiences of relatives and carers, we will highlight some key differences between existing approaches to working with relatives and the PCT-informed approach that we are proposing. The chapter concludes with a case study and a discussion of how PCT principles might be applied in clinical practice.

Terminology

A quick note on the language used in this chapter. For the sake of brevity, we use the term 'relative' to refer to anyone who has a close personal relationship and a significant amount of contact with someone who is accessing support from secondary mental health services. This might be a family member, romantic partner, or close friend. Relative, in this context, might refer to someone who is defined as a 'carer' for the person using mental health services (and we sometimes use this term), but this is not necessarily the case. We recognise that people who might be defined as relatives and carers are a heterogenous population with diverse backgrounds, experiences, and personal circumstances. Our aim with this chapter, however, is to make it as relevant and useful to the largest group possible.

DOI: 10.4324/9781003041344-7

Experiences of relatives

There is now a great deal of evidence to suggest that providing care for someone who is experiencing mental health difficulties is frequently a demanding and distressing experience (Brown & Birtwistle, 1998; Kuipers et al., 2010). There is also evidence that this can have a significant impact on the health and wellbeing of relatives. Compared to the general population, relatives appear to be at an increased risk of experiencing their own mental health problems (Onwumere et al., 2016; Sin et al., 2021). They are more likely to reach diagnostic threshold for a range of psychiatric disorders such as post-traumatic stress disorder, depression, and anxiety (Barton & Jackson, 2008). Relatives are also more likely to report higher rates of social isolation and lower levels of quality of life (Hayes et al., 2015). Relatives often neglect their own hobbies and interests, have their employment prospects curtailed, and experience various other economic disadvantages (Lippi, 2016). As well as playing a potentially important role in supporting people who experience mental health difficulties, relatives contribute to huge financial savings for society. One report, for example, estimated that family members who are supporting people diagnosed with psychosis spectrum disorders saved the UK economy £1.25 billion per year, mainly through the provision of unpaid care (Schizophrenia Commission, 2012). It is imperative, therefore, that mental health services carefully consider how they can support the health and wellbeing of relatives.

This raises the question of why so many relatives continue to act as carers, despite the impact this can have on their health and personal circumstances. While relatives report multiple challenges associated with having a family member who requires support from secondary mental healthcare, there is also evidence to suggest that there are some positive or rewarding aspects to this experience. Relatives in one qualitative study, for example, reported that their family member's experience with first-episode psychosis had brought them closer together and deepened their relationship (McCann et al., 2011). One participant reported:

> The good thing, I think, is that this experience has got me closer to him because before this we didn't talk much. As any boy who is a teenager, they don't talk to the parents and even less to their mother because it's embarrassing to be seen talking to their mother.
>
> (McCann et al., 2011, p. 384)

A recent systematic review of qualitative literature relating to the experiences of caregivers for people diagnosed withs schizophrenia identified a range of positive impacts of caring, including increased family solidarity, self-confidence, personal growth, and affection towards their relative (Shiraishi & Reilly, 2019).

From a PCT perspective, it seems likely that relatives continue to provide care and maintain relationships of this kind, despite the associated challenges, because they have higher-level goals relating to their relationship with the family member who is reporting mental health difficulties. Examples of higher-level goals might include 'be a good father', 'be a supportive partner', or 'keep my child safe'. Meeting these higher-level goals, however, will sometimes disrupt other important personal goals for relatives. Goals that might be disrupted or impaired by being a carer might include 'succeed in my career', 'live a healthy life', or 'engage in hobbies I enjoy'. Consequently, relatives are likely to experience some intra-psychic conflict between goals relating to their relationship with their family member and other personally meaningful goals. As we have seen in previous chapters, being in a state of conflict disrupts people's capacity to effectively control important perceptual variables. This chapter aims to both explore the kinds of conflicts that relatives can experience, and consider how they can be supported by mental health services to resolve these.

Before considering the unique contribution that PCT might bring to understanding and addressing problems in personal relationships between patients and relatives, we will first consider existing theoretical frameworks and approaches in this area.

Existing approaches to working with relatives

Many different approaches to working with the relatives of people experiencing mental health difficulties have been developed and evaluated. Much of the work in this area has focused on improving outcomes for people reporting psychosis-related difficulties or who have received a diagnosis of schizophrenia. Two of the most widely implemented approaches to family intervention are behavioural family therapy (BFT) and cognitive behavioural family intervention (CBT-FI). BFT, which was developed by Ian Falloon and colleagues, aims to reduce relapse risk by developing the stress-management capacity of the patient and their family (Falloon, 2015; Falloon et al., 1982). This is achieved, it is argued, by developing people's understanding of 'mental illness' and through the use of behavioural approaches to develop family members' problem-solving skills. CBT-FI also uses psychoeducation materials, along with facilitated family discussions, to help family members develop alternative appraisals of their experiences, improve communication between family members, and gain new problem solving and coping strategies, with the aim of reducing relapse (Barrowclough & Tarrier, 1997; Kuipers et al., 2002). A systematic review of family interventions concluded that they might reduce relapse rates and hospitalisations, but the poor methodological quality of studies could have resulted in an overestimation of their effectiveness (Pharoah et al., 2010). Common to many approaches to family work is the idea of reducing relapses by addressing issues relating to 'expressed emotion', which is a construct that we will now explore in more depth.

The concept of 'expressed emotion'

Classic studies conducted by George W. Brown and colleagues in the 1950s and 1960s appeared to show that people diagnosed with schizophrenia who were discharged from hospital to their family home were at higher risk of subsequent readmission than those who were discharged to other kinds of accommodation, such as supported housing (Brown et al., 1962, 1972). The emotional atmosphere within the home was offered as an explanation for this apparently counterintuitive finding. Counterintuitive, because it might be assumed that returning to your family home would lead to improved outcomes compared to living away from relatives in supported housing. Home environments where communication between relatives was characterised by critical comments, hostility, or emotional over-involvement were referred to as having high levels of 'expressed emotion' (Amaresha & Venkatasubramanian, 2012). The idea of high expressed emotion has informed much of the thinking about how mental health services should approach their work with the relatives. It has been applied to people who have been diagnosed with a variety of disorders, including schizophrenia, depression, and bipolar affective disorder (Amaresha & Venkatasubramanian, 2012; Hayhurst et al., 1997; Kim & Miklowitz, 2004).

The stress-vulnerability model

Why should it be the case, however, that critical or hostile comments from family members would necessarily lead someone to experience worse mental health outcomes? Similarly, what is it about having a relative who is 'emotionally over-involved' that is so deeply problematic? Proponents of the expressed emotion hypothesis argue the effects of familial interactions of this kind are deleterious because they create an environmental stressor that can result in 'relapse' amongst people reporting mental health difficulties (Amaresha & Venkatasubramanian, 2012). Expressed emotion, therefore, is placed within a stress-vulnerability framework for understanding mental health difficulties. High expressed emotion is a problem because it creates stress. Because of patients 'inherited vulnerabilities', it is argued, this stress increases the likelihood of them experiencing a relapse. It is worth explaining this stress-vulnerability model of 'psychopathology' in more detail.

The stress-vulnerability model (or stress-diathesis model as it is sometimes referred to) developed by Zubin and Spring (1977) attempted to integrate the prevailing biological, ecological, and behavioural, aetiological models of schizophrenia that were available at that time. Biological models proposed that problems with health, including mental health, were the product of an individual's genetic predisposition. Ecological models saw the problems experienced by people diagnosed with schizophrenia as arising from their environmental conditions. Behavioural models were concerned with the role that learning and development played in the development of psychological difficulties. Zubin and Spring (1977), however, proposed that people possess a degree of 'vulnerability', and, under certain circumstances, this will result in the individual experiencing an episode of schizophrenia. Vulnerability, according to this model, arises from a combination of genetic factors and life events (exposure to disease or traumatic events, for example). While Zubin and Spring's (1977) stress-diathesis model was originally developed as an aetiological model of schizophrenia, it has since been applied to other diagnostic categories (e.g., Goh & Agius, 2010; Kim & Chung, 2014).

Distinctions between Perceptual Control Theory and existing theories and approaches

A PCT understanding of the difficulties that can occur in personal relationships, and how these difficulties relate to an individual's mental health, deviates significantly from explanations that rely on constructs such as expressed emotion or stress-vulnerability. Prior to exploring these differences, we will consider some areas of apparent similarity. PCT corresponds with Zubin and Spring's (1977) hypothesis that the environment in which an individual exists is an important consideration when trying to understand behaviour, and that mental health difficulties can only be understood when we consider the interaction between factors that are both inside and outside of the person. As with PCT, Zubin and Spring (1977) also place their model within a homeostatic framework, arguing that when a person is exposed to stress, 'adaptive capacities' come into play that seek to counteract this stress and return the person to a state of contentment. Where adaptations are unable to cope with the stress placed upon the system, they argue, this results in the occurrence of psychiatric disorders. PCT is also consistent with principles of homeostasis, arguing that people seek to control their perceptions to maintain them in line with internally specified reference values.

There are some important differences, however, between PCT and the stress-vulnerability model. From a PCT perspective, there are several problems with the utility of the stress-vulnerability model as a means for understanding psychological distress.

The first problem, from our perspective, is less with what the model proposes as much as it concerns the kind of model that is being proposed. The stress-vulnerability model, as with virtually all models in the mental health literature, is purely conceptual in nature. In contrast, PCT provides a conceptual framework together with a functional mode. Functional models, elsewhere called computational or generative models (Guest & Martin, 2021), aim to simulate the phenomenon they seek to explain. The advantage of this approach is that it constrains the theory builder to concepts that can be stated mathematically, implemented in computer code, and run as simulations. This allows for a more transparent approach to theory building and testing. Models that are solely verbally or conceptually conceived are much more open to misinterpretation and, further, cannot be tested in the same manner. The key concept of PCT – that humans control a hierarchy level of perceptions – has been tested in a series of studies comparing observed data with functional models (Parker et al., 2020). Whilst these studies have focused on lower-level perceptions of object motion, it is conceivable that higher perceptions of principles, such as ‘honesty’ or ‘care’, can be investigated in the same transparent, rigorous manner. In contrast, the stress-vulnerability model has never been investigated using computational or functional models and, indeed, this approach has not been applied to other similar theories. PCT is distinguished from other theories by its description of the hypothesised existence of the controlled perception, which provides a powerful means of applying a functional modelling approach to science in a field that, thus far, seems distant from it.

The second issue relates the stress-diathesis model's underlying assumptions about the nature of living things. The stress-diathesis model is, essentially, linear in nature. According to Zubin and Spring's (1977) model, ‘stress’, however that construct is defined, impacts on the individual concerned, and this results in them experiencing symptoms of psychopathology. This assumption of linear causality informs many current approaches to family work, including BFT and CBT-FI. Rather than linear causality, however, PCT is underpinned by an assumption of circular causality. Runkel (2007, p. 85) explains the concept of circular causality in this way:

> The key idea in circular causality is that the internal causes and causes from the environment operate simultaneously, not sequentially, not in tandem or in episodes. The internal operations affect what will be perceived from the environment, and what is perceived affects what is done internally, and all that goes on continuously and seamlessly.

So, from a PCT perspective, what are described as ‘stressors’ in the stress-vulnerability model could be understood as disturbances that, if left unchecked, would disrupt the state of variables currently being controlled by an individual. Through the process of control, individual's act against these disturbances to neutralise their effects and maintain important perceptual variables in their desired state. Rather than these steps occurring sequentially, however, the process of control is a synchronous and uninterrupted process whereby the person's actions change the state of a variable to keep it in line with reference values held for the state of that perception.

We will try to highlight some of the key differences between PCT and the stress-vulnerability model with a hypothetical example. John is man in his twenties who has been given a diagnosis of schizophrenia. He is living at his parents' home and is being supported by his local community mental health team. John reports that he is hearing voices telling him that he will be harmed if leaves the house. He also says that he is feeling depressed and struggles to motivate himself to do everyday tasks. John's parents, however, have become frustrated with the fact that he is not looking for paid work and does not help with chores around the home. One day, tensions come to a head and his father shouts at him, 'You're a total waste of space! Why don't you do something useful for a change?' John is upset by his father's outburst and angrily storms out of the house. John's father is also saddened by the exchange and feels remorseful about becoming angry with his son.

From the perspective of the stress-vulnerability model, this could be understood as a situation where John has been exposed to a source of environmental stress: his father's critical comments. The model would argue that stressful incidents, such as the one described, risk exacerbating John's problems with voice hearing, depression, and low motivation. The focus of mental health support, from this perspective, is likely to involve efforts to reduce the overall levels of 'expressed emotion' within the home to minimise the levels of stress that John is encountering. The care team involved might try and achieve this by using psychoeducation and cognitive-behavioural techniques to encourage his parents to reappraise John's lack of activity as resulting from his mental health difficulties, and to increase his parent's ability to cope with this difficult situation. This strategy would be consistent with many current approaches to family work.

The PCT explanation of this scenario would be rather different. From this perspective, calling someone 'a waste of space' would only be problematic for the person if this statement acted as a disturbance to a perceptual variable that they were attempting to control. If someone had a goal to 'be a productive person', or 'be a good son', or 'live a worthwhile life', for example, such a comment could potentially make it difficult for the person to control perceptions relating to those goals in a satisfactory way. If someone were not concerned about being called a 'waste of space' by a particular person, this would not act as a disturbance and, therefore, it is unlikely the comment would cause any significant distress. This possibility has been tested in a study where people were presented with descriptions of themselves that contradicted their self-concept (Robertson et al., 1999). The findings were consistent with the expectation that statements about people are corrected when inconsistent with their self-concept and ignored otherwise, supporting the notion that people control a perception of their self-concept, and this controlling is evident in social interactions.

We can infer from John's response – becoming angry and storming out – that his father's comments did indeed disturb a variable that was currently being controlled by John. With such limited information about the scenario in question, it is not possible to say exactly what variable (or variables) John is controlling. It is not always easy to infer what someone is controlling for merely by observing their behaviour (Willett et al., 2017). For the sake of this example, however, let us imagine that the variable being controlled relates to John's perception of the quality of the relationship with his father. Perhaps his goal is to 'maintain a good relationship with my dad'. Being called 'a waste of space', in this situation, might well disrupt John's ability to maintain that goal within acceptable parameters.

If John's only concern were to maintain a good quality relationship with his father, however, why doesn't he simply carry out the household tasks that have become such a bone of contention? Similarly, if John's father is remorseful about the exchange with his son, what was it that prompted him to act in such an angry manner? This suggests that there is something else happening which we have not yet considered in relation to this situation. It seems likely that there are several other relevant goals that both John and his father are controlling for; goals that they themselves might not yet have had the opportunity to consider fully. PCT provides a theoretical framework for understanding complex interactions, such as this one, and offers some suggestions for how difficulties in relationships can be addressed.

Applying PCT principles of control, conflict, and reorganisation

The PCT approach replaces terms such as 'expressed emotion' and 'stress vulnerability' with terms that describe principles that permeate everyday life to varying degrees – control, conflict, and reorganisation. These principles are not specific to people with mental health issues and their relatives. To put it simply, we all attempt to control aspects of our selves, others, and the world that matter to us to varying degrees, and for some people and their relatives, this entails conflict because of the overlaps in what is being controlled and the tenacity and effort with which it is being controlled. The solution to ongoing conflict is awareness – the capacity to 'take a step back' and notice what people are attempting to control, where this entails conflict, what the goals might be 'above' the conflict, and to considering this whole situation in enough depth and detail to generate, often spontaneously, a new perspective on the problem.

Thus, any difficult interaction between people that raises 'stress' for a sustained period can be understood as two or more conflicting control systems. 'Overinvolvement' or 'overprotection' may be the words used to describe interactions in which a carer or relative is trying to try to control for what they think the patient wants or needs, such as to never let them leave the neighbourhood by themselves to prevent them being assaulted again. In PCT, these terms are only ever references for the perceptual variables concerning involvement or protection – what is over-involved or over-protective can only be defined from the person experiencing some level of these that is not at the desired state. Conflict is evident when patient and relative's views on how much protection or involvement is warranted differs from both their references and they strive to correct it. This striving would be observed by others as arguments or tension. Thus, if the patient actually wants to leave the neighbourhood to make new friends, or to find a job, this generates conflict because it disturbs their relative's perception of the extent to which they can protect or care for them. We can also use techniques informed by PCT, such as the Method of Levels (MOL; Carey, 2006) approach described in Chapter 4, to explore the level 'above' the perception of protectivity. What is particularly important for the relative about keeping the patient safe? What experience are they actually trying to create or sustain? It might be easily assumed that the experience they are trying to maintain is the ongoing survival of their relative. But is this the case? Gentle, curious questioning may reveal that, actually, the relative is trying to keep memories of the death of their husband out of their awareness, or maybe the fear is of a serious injury like the one that their own father experienced whilst the relative was a child.

We can also take a PCT approach to explore 'criticism' in more depth. As explained earlier, criticism would be 'stressful' to the extent that it opposed a goal for a trait that the patient tries to maintain – such as when a person who wants to be kind is told they are 'nasty'. Yet, criticism may often not be intentional on the part of the relative. It may be a subgoal (further down the hierarchy) to support another goal, such as the goal of protection described above. It may take some time of exploration with the relative before they realise why they get so critical. For some people it might be a way to keep their patient's confidence low enough that they don't take unnecessary risks. For others it might be an attempt to stop reminding themselves of their own perceived inadequacies in life.

A further step is hostility. Again, this is rarely a goal in itself. Hostility, whether intentional or not, is a means to another end. In fact, models of control systems in conflict consistently show that the outputs of both systems increase (McClelland, 1994). Think of the 'output' in this case as the volume of voice, increased gesticulation of behaviour and more extreme emotional facial expression, and the heart rate increase to support this escalation. Thus, from a PCT perspective, hostility can be seen as emerging dynamically from conflict rather than as a 'trigger' of 'stress'.

Because we are discussing terms such as 'criticism' and 'hostility', at this point it is worth highlighting another key distinction between PCT and other approaches to working with families. At issue is the matter of who defines interactions as being critical or hostile, or who gets to make the final judgement about whether a relative is 'emotionally overinvolved' with a patient. Typically, these constructs have been assessed using outcome measures such as the Camberwell Family Interview (Vaughn & Leff, 1976), where a recorded interview with a family member is reviewed by a practitioner or researcher who rates 'observed emotions', such as 'warmth' or 'hostility', and counts the number of comments that are judged to be either 'positive' or 'critical'. From a PCT perspective, however, what is important is the first-person perspective of the individual concerned, and this is prioritised over the perspective of third-party observers. Whether a comment is experienced as critical can only be judged from the perspective of the person who is on the receiving end of the comment. Indeed, someone might make a comment that is intended to be complimentary, but which is experienced as a criticism by the other person. Similarly, whether a relative is emotionally over-, under-, or optimally involved cannot be accurately judged by an external observer (although they may well have opinions on this topic).

It is actually possible to draw upon models of control systems to appreciate how other phenomena we see in families can emerge from the dynamics of conflict. Appreciating this takes the blame away from pointing at whose behaviour caused what level of stress, and which unwanted outcome. The whole process is an interactive system that deserves to be understood from a higher level. Computational models of conflict show two important phenomena: stalemates and oscillations (McClelland, 2022). These are the two most common difficulties experienced in families with patients coming for treatment – being 'stuck' in terms of lack of progress, loss of motivation, or reduced emotional expressivity – and 'losing control', which might manifest as escalating arguments, panic attacks, or episodes of psychosis. The practitioner who reminds themselves of these facts about systems in conflict can keep a steady perspective, and, through even-handed exploration, begin to foster this perspective in patients and their relatives. Blaming the patient, blaming the relative, blaming the brain, blaming the medication aren't simply unpleasant; they are incomplete and inaccurate explanations of what is going on. The clinician strives to promote a fuller understanding in themselves and others, but also knows this is unachievable because the control dynamics are regularly changing. This makes genuine curiosity the only feasible, lasting attitude that a clinician can return to. They need to seek extra supervision when their authentic curiosity about a patient and their relatives feels out of reach, and work on building a perspective that allows it to return.

Illustrative case study

To illustrate these points with an example, Vignette 7.1 presents a case study of a conflict between Alice and Sophia, who are mother and daughter.

Applying PCT in practice

Because every family situation is different, rather than offering prescriptive advice about the precise steps practitioners should adopt in this kind of scenario, we will instead offer some general PCT-informed principles that are designed to be applied to a range of situations that involve conflicts between family members. The principles and processes have been described previously in the context of how a professional mediator may support negotiation and compromise between two conflicting parties, such as during legal disputes and international negotiations (McClelland & Mansell, 2019), and are of relevance here.

Vignette 7.1 Conflict between family members

Sophia is 26 years old. She has returned to live with her mother, Alice, after a recent admission to an acute mental health inpatient unit. Prior to her admission, Sophia had been living independently in her own accommodation. Although she has experienced some improvements in her mental health, Sophia continues to report that she feels paranoid. Her main concern is that she is being constantly watched by hidden cameras. This makes Sophia feel anxious most of the time, and this becomes much worse whenever she is in other people's company. She has found that her concerns about being monitored are less troubling when she spends time alone in her bedroom, where she says she feels safer. Sophia also reports that smoking cannabis makes her feel more relaxed and less paranoid. As such, Sophia spends most of her day in her bedroom smoking cannabis and only leaves for short periods of time, generally to buy more cannabis when she runs out.

Alice is concerned about the amount of time Sophia is spending on her own and worries that her cannabis use is making her mental health problems worse. She is concerned that Sophia is not socialising with her friends, engaging in hobbies or pastimes, or looking for work. Alice is also frustrated that Sophia is trying to avoid meeting with the staff from the Early Intervention in Psychosis team who are seeking to provide her with support. This has become a major source of tension between Sophia and Alice. For several days, Alice has been trying to encourage Sophia to leave her bedroom to engage in activities and meet with her mental health team, but her attempts have not been successful. Disagreements between Sophia and Alice result in them having daily arguments.

When the staff from the mental health team next visit, Sophia and Alice are both visibly distressed. Sophia says that her mother is 'driving me mad' with the pressure she is putting on her. Meanwhile, Alice says the stress of the situation is affecting her physical health, and she has had to take time off work as a result. Alice and Sophia say that their constant arguing is ruining their relationship, which they both find upsetting.

Explore sources of interpersonal conflict

Figure 7.1 provides a diagrammatic representation of the situation described in Box 7.1. The 'node' of conflict between Alice and Sophia is the amount of conflict that Sophia has with other people. This is represented at the bottom of the diagram. In PCT terms, the amount of contact between Sophia and other people is referred to as the 'controlled variable'. This conflict is occurring

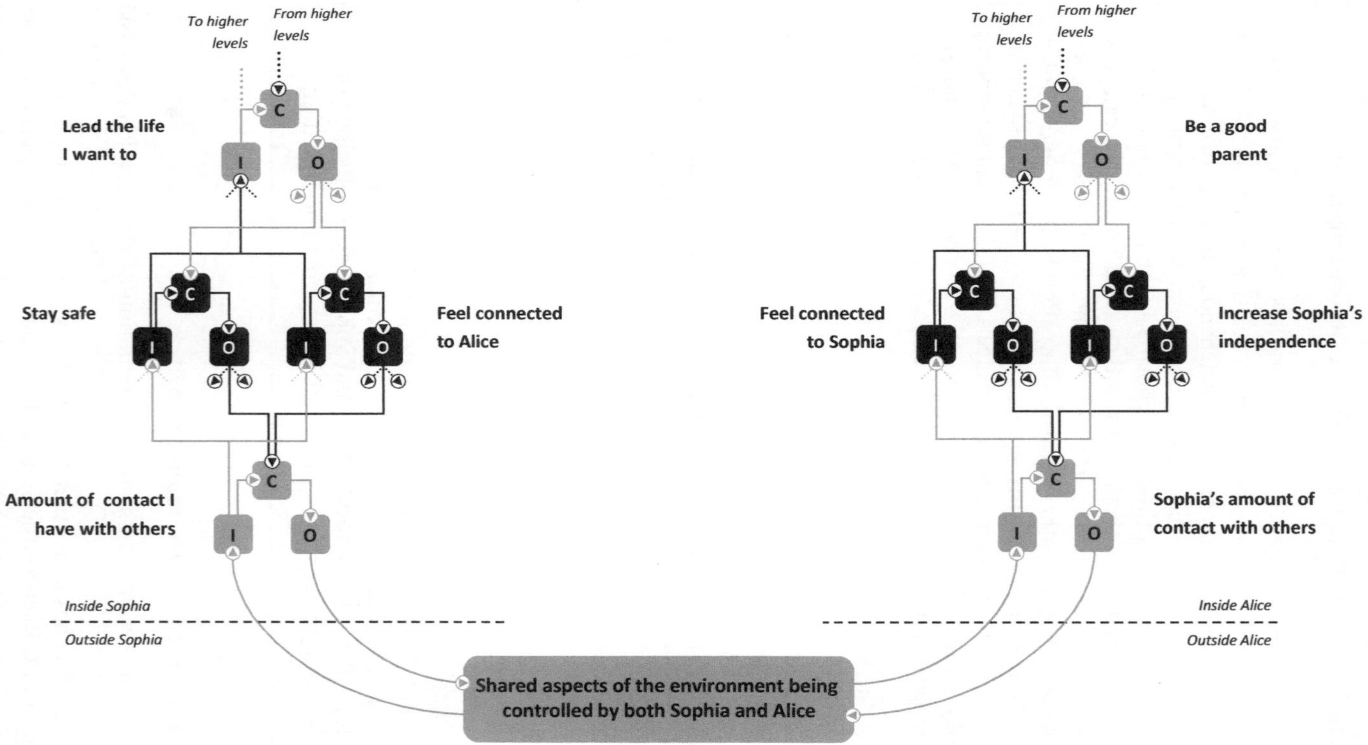

Figure 7.1 Diagram illustrating an interpersonal conflict between Sophia (the patient) and Alice (the parent) relating to the amount of contact between Sophia and other people. The diagram also includes intrapersonal conflicts experienced by both Sophia and Alice relating to the control of this variable.

because Alice and Sophia have different goals for the state of this controlled variable. Alice's control over this variable is acting as a disturbance to Sophia's controlling, and vice versa. To understand and resolve this conflict, it is necessary to explore Alice and Sophia's higher-level goals that are relevant to this controlled variable. Once an interpersonal conflict is identified, the goal of the PCT-informed practitioner is to try and clarify the higher-level goals of the individuals concerned. Interpersonal conflicts will only persist in situations where someone is also in a state of intrapersonal conflict.

To illustrate why it is necessarily the case that interpersonal conflicts only arise in the context of intrapersonal conflicts, one straightforward solution to resolving the disagreement between Alice and Sophia would be for them to stop having contact with each other altogether. If they did not spend any time in each other's company, it would not be possible for them to disagree and argue with each other. Presumably, Alice and Sophia continue to have contact because they each have goals relating to the quality of their relationship, which means that ceasing to see each other is not an option for them. This means that they are in a state of conflict. Resolving interpersonal conflicts, therefore, requires the resolution of relevant intrapersonal conflicts.

Exploring intrapersonal conflicts

On the bottom left-hand side of the diagram in Figure 7.1, we can see that Sophia has a lower-level control system that relates to the 'amount of contact I have with others'. An input function (marked 'I' in the diagram) produces a signal specifying the current state of perceptual inputs for this control system. This signal then passes to a comparator function (marked 'C'). Perceptual input is compared to the reference value for the desired state of this variable. Where there is a difference between the state of a perception and its corresponding reference value, this will create an error signal. Error in this case does not mean 'bad' or 'wrong'. Instead, it just means that there is a difference between the current perception of a variable and the reference value specifying the desired state of that variable. This error signal passes to the output function (marked 'O'), which produces an output signal. At this lowest level in the perceptual hierarchy, this will lead Sophia to adjust her behaviour, with the goal of bringing current perceptions in line with her reference values. Crucially, reference values are set by the outputs of higher-level control systems. To understand Sophia's current predicament, therefore, we need to travel further up the perceptual hierarchy.

Going up levels

The next level up has two control systems that conflict with each other. One has a goal relating to 'staying safe', whereas the other has a goal to 'feel connected to Alice'. Currently, these goals are incompatible. The more Sophia tries to meet her 'staying safe' goal – by, for example, staying in her bedroom, avoiding other people, and smoking cannabis – the more this creates problems in her relationship with her mother. If, however, she tries to meet her goal to 'feel connected to Alice', maybe by leaving her room and socialising with others, the more error she is creating with her 'stay safe' goal. If we travel to the highest level depicted in Sophia's perceptual hierarchy, we can see she has a high-level goal to 'lead the life I want'. It is this higher-level control system that is setting the incompatible goals for lower levels.

If we look at the right side of the diagram, we can see that Alice is also in a state of conflict. Her lower-level goal relates to the amount of contact that Sophia is having with other people. At the mid-level, Alice has two conflicted goals: 'feel connected to Sophia' and 'increase Sophia's independence'. At present, meeting one of these goals is impeding her ability to meet the other. Alice's efforts to increase Sophia's independence – by encouraging her to leave her room and meet with the mental health team, for example – are negatively impacting on the quality of her relationship with her daughter. At the highest level, which is setting the incompatible reference values, Alice's goal is to 'be a good parent'.

For Alice and Sophia, continuing to experience these unresolved conflicts is likely to be distressing. In this situation, one outcome is to oscillate between reducing error on either side of the conflict, but this will have the effect of increasing error for the other control system. Alternatively, Alice and Sophia could meet just one of their goals at the expense of the other. Sophia could sacrifice the quality of her relationship with Alice by just attending to the 'stay safe' goal. Neither solution (oscillating between goals or only attending to one side of the conflict) is likely to be satisfactory, however, because Alice and Sophia will remain in a state of chronic, unresolved conflict. This is likely to be distressing and will maintain the ongoing interpersonal conflict. What is required to resolve this situation is a change to the higher-level goals that are setting the incompatible reference values for lower-level control systems.

Facilitating reorganisation

As outlined in Chapter 2, the proposed mechanism of change in PCT is called reorganisation. Practitioners can support the process of reorganisation by helping people to shift their awareness onto the level that is setting the incompatible reference values for lower-level goals. The Method of Levels (MOL), which is described in Chapter 4, is one way of achieving this. Looking for indications that someone's awareness has momentarily drifted onto potentially relevant background thoughts, and then asking about this, is one way of helping people to move their awareness towards higher-level goals. If Sophia and Alice can sustain their awareness on their high-level goals – 'live the life I want to' and 'be a good parent', respectively – then this could support the reorganisation process and lead to helpful new perspectives on the problems they are encountering.

For Alice, it might be helpful for her to reflect on what being a good parent looks like from her perspective, to consider how she is currently working towards this goal, and whether there are other ways to think about being a good parent. This could provide Alice with the opportunity to develop a new perspective on 'being a good parent'. Through the process of reorganisation, it is possible that this new perspective does not create conflict at lower levels of the hierarchy. Similarly, Sophia might find it helpful to reflect on what 'leading the life I want to' means to her and whether there are different ways of thinking about this. It might also be helpful for Alice and Sophia to reflect on areas of agreement between them. Feeling connected with each other is something that is important to them both. It might be that there are other ways of maintaining their connection that do not conflict with other important goals that they are both trying to meet.

Because reorganisation is a random trial-and-error system, it is not possible to say what solutions might emerge from the process of Alice and Sophia exploring higher-level goals. Potentially, however, the sensitive exploration of high-level goals could lead to the resolution of intrapersonal conflicts, which, in turn, could lead to the cessation of interpersonal conflicts.

Adopt a stance of genuine curiosity

Although we have some information about Sophia and Alice's predicament, the goal of the PCT-informed practitioner in this situation is to try and avoid offering advice or suggestions about how they should resolve their difficulties. Instead, as in MOL, questions are asked with a genuine sense of curiosity. Asking questions in this way provides opportunities for Alice and Sophia to sustain their awareness on aspects of the problem that they might not have had the opportunity to explore in depth before. This process will enable everyone involved to gain a much richer understanding of their own goals, the goals of other people, and will support the process of reorganisation.

While practitioners are encouraged to avoid giving unsolicited advice, it might well be appropriate to offer information that is relevant to the family's situation. Passing on details about a peer support group for carers might be an example of useful information to provide Alice. Telling Alice that she should, 'definitely attend the group because you would really benefit from the support on offer', would be an example of the kind of advice that is unlikely to be helpful. Where possible, practitioners should focus on providing family members with potentially useful information and aim to minimise the extent to which they attempt to encourage, persuade, or cajole people to take one course of action over another. The aim is to create an environment where people can generate their own bespoke solutions to the problems that they are encountering.

Provide a context where people can speak openly

It has been argued, from a PCT perspective, that what defines the 'therapeutic relationship' is the degree to which people feel able to speak openly about whatever is on their mind, without filtering or censoring the content of their thoughts (Carey et al., 2012). This creates a context where people can explore higher level goals, and the conflicts they give rise to, facilitating the reorganisation process. Unlike some approaches, which stipulate exactly which family members should be present for family therapy to be successful, a PCT approach would require practitioners to adopt a flexible approach to creating contexts where people can resolve intrapersonal and interpersonal conflicts. In the case of Alice and Sophia, it might be that they find it helpful to meet to discuss the difficulties they are encountering in their relationship. It might also be the case, however, that one or both feels inhibited about openly expressing what is on their mind in front of the other. Out of a fear of upsetting or angering the other, for example. As much as possible, the practitioner's goal is to try and facilitate a context that is considered satisfactory by both parties.

Hope and optimism

We were fortunate enough to have Dr David Shiers review an early version of this chapter. David is a retired general practitioner and carer for his daughter, who experiences psychosis. He has been instrumental in the development of early intervention in psychosis services in the United Kingdom. After reading the draft chapter, David commented that one of the most troubling aspects of his initial contact with mental health services was the pessimistic view of some health professionals about his daughter's prospects. Within the language used by these professionals, David detected an implicit message that his daughter's mental health condition and level of functioning would inexorably decline. From his perspective, the 'therapeutic optimism' that he experienced from other mental health professionals and services was much more helpful and instilled a sense of hope about his daughter's future. In our discussion about this chapter, David wondered whether PCT had anything to say about the topics of 'hope' and 'therapeutic optimism'. From our perspective, inherent within PCT is an assumption that growth and change are inevitable features of human life. The innate reorganisation system, which enables us to generate new perspectives on problems and resolve conflicts, makes humans highly adept at responding to life's challenges and changing circumstances. Health professionals who are informed by PCT, therefore, are aware that, in the right circumstances, people are capable of generating novel solutions to resolve seemingly intractable problems. Reorganisation cannot be directed or forced to find solutions – patience and sustained optimism are essential for people to fully explore conflicts and allow reorganisation to occur where it is most helpful. This acknowledges that change is not a linear process. It may feel challenging when optimism is hard to come by and solutions seem distant. It encourages practitioners to remain alongside people, with an attitude of patience and optimism that they will, eventually, find more helpful perspectives on what is concerning, bothering, or distressing them. PCT-informed practice takes a stance of being there for the full haul, whether it be short or long. As such, PCT offers a profoundly hopeful view of people's capacity for change and growth.

In Reflection 7.1, Pru, who is the mother of Jasmine Waldorf, one of the authors of this book, describes an experience she encountered whilst trying to support Jasmine during a period of crisis. Pru describes how her ability to control factors that she saw as important – such as Jasmine's physical and mental health, the kind of care her daughter was being offered, and the quality of her relationship with Jasmine – was impaired by the nature of the environment (a busy Accident and Emergency Department) and the approach taken by the healthcare professionals involved. Pru concludes by reflecting on the kind of approach that she thinks would have been more helpful for her (and also for Jasmine) in the situation. Central to the approach described by Pru is the aim of seeking to establish the goals of everyone involved in these kinds of situations (patients, relatives, and staff), and creating a context where people can express themselves calmly and openly to inform shared decision making.

Reflection 7.1 Pru's experience of supporting Jasmine

The experience of relatives is perhaps best illustrated by the way services operate at crisis points. One such crisis point came for my daughter Jasmine and I when the services seemed to be offering a choice. The care team (who were Accident and Emergency Department (A&E) doctors – none of her team were present) suggested that I work with them and persuade Jasmine that she should take part in a medical assessment. Alternatively, the outcome would be that the police officers would need to step in and take responsibility for the situation, and Jasmine would be 'sectioned' under the Mental Health Act (1983) against her will. Neither option seemed suitable to me. Both seemed to come with obvious drawbacks. Jasmine and I disagreed on what was best at that moment in time. I thought that Jasmine was in dire need of urgent care, but her perception was different, she felt that care wasn't needed. And she felt that I was betraying her and not supporting her wishes in pressurising her to agree to being observed by healthcare professionals (this involved taking blood for a blood test and giving her treatment because she had been complaining of a pain in her abdomen).

The hospital staff saw Jasmine and me as a mother and child. They seemed to hold a bias that it's a mother's duty to 'do the right thing' and persuade their child to be compliant, and that their 'expert wishes' should be followed at any cost. But I saw it differently, we were two adults trying to do what's best. We were both depleted after no sleep or rest, weary from waiting for hours for help. No relative should be faced with responsibility when in that state of mind. But even if I'd been at my strongest, I wouldn't have been able to persuade Jasmine, without coercing, and ultimately, misleading her into a situation that she didn't want to happen. That would be a betrayal of trust. So, the choice wasn't really a choice in the end. I couldn't be the pivotal person or sole decision maker in that situation and was there alone – her care coordinator refused to attend in support of Jasmine, and I was unable to reach the out of hours team. I felt we needed space and a calm environment to create a solution together, and to reduce the sense of stress and emergency. It was all making the situation worse as it was causing fear and alarm in Jasmine, who, at that time, was experiencing some confusion from hearing voices and seeing visual disturbances. However, we weren't given the resources to do this. We were in a crowded A&E lobby, with no privacy, and people all around us staring as this massive drama played out. It was dreadful.

What I needed in that situation was a chance for everyone to be asked what they wanted. For us to be met in a calm and considered way with kindness. Services need to meet patients and relatives on their own terms to begin with. This takes time and is obstructed by an attitude of urgency, stress, fear, and an 'emergency'-like response. It prevents the necessary time for relatives to support decision making. Supported decision making requires that services explain options to service users to help them weigh up the pros and cons. Relatives should be given full information about what care entails so there is informed consent. However, too often, there is a pressure to make a rapid decision. On some occasions a rapid decision can and should be made. But flexibility is essential at this point for people to create the episode of care they need for their relatives and what we needed was to de-escalate the situation and some quiet time and space to discuss things rather than pressure from police and A&E doctors.

Summary

In this chapter, we have sought to outline the unique contribution that PCT could bring to working with the families of people using secondary mental healthcare. We have highlighted some important areas of distinction – both theoretical and practical – between a PCT-informed approach to working with families and existing approaches. Rather than conceptualising the difficulties that can occur in families within a 'stress-vulnerability' framework, or as arising from high levels of 'expressed emotion', we have argued that the universal PCT principles of control, conflict, and reorganisation are sufficient for understanding and addressing problems of this kind. We have also emphasised the importance of seeking to understand problems within close personal relationships from a first-person perspective rather than from the perspective of the observer. Finally, we have offered some suggestions for practitioners on how they might use PCT principles to work more effectively with relatives and patients to help them address problems in their relationships. We have argued that supporting the resolution of intrapersonal conflicts is central to the question of how people resolve distressing interpersonal conflicts. Although research informed by PCT in this area is currently in its infancy, we believe that it offers a powerful theoretical framework for developing approaches to working with relatives which could make an important difference to the health and wellbeing of relatives and patients.

References

Amaresha, A. C., & Venkatasubramanian, G. (2012). Expressed emotion in schizophrenia: An overview. In *Indian Journal of Psychological Medicine*, *34*(1), 12–20. https://doi.org/10.4103/0253-7176.96149

Barrowclough, C., & Tarrier, N. (1997). *Families of schizophrenic patients: Cognitive behavioural intervention*. Stanley Thornes.

Barton, K., & Jackson, C. (2008). Reducing symptoms of trauma among carers of people with psychosis: Pilot study examining the impact of writing about caregiving experiences. *Australian and New Zealand Journal of Psychiatry*, *42*(8). https://doi.org/10.1080/00048670802203434

Brown, G. W., Birley, J. L., & Wing, J. K. (1972). Influence of family life on the course of schizophrenic disorders: A replication. *British Journal of Psychiatry*, *121*(562), 241–258. https://doi.org/10.1192/bjp.121.3.241

Brown, G. W., Monk, E. M., Carstairs, G. M., & Wing, J. K. (1962). Influence of family life on the course of schizophrenic illness. *British Journal of Psychiatry*, *16*(2), 55–68.

Brown, S., & Birtwistle, J. (1998). People with schizophrenia and their families: Fifteen-year outcome. *British Journal of Psychiatry*, *173*, 139–144. https://doi.org/10.1192/bjp.173.2.139

Carey, T. A. (2006). *The Method of Levels: How to do psychotherapy without getting in the way*. Living Control Systems Publishing.

Carey, T., Kelly, R., Mansell, W., & Tai, S. (2012). What's therapeutic about the therapeutic relationship? A hypothesis for practice informed by Perceptual Control Theory. *The Cognitive Behaviour Therapist*, *5*(2–3), 47–59. doi:10.1017/S1754470X12000037

Falloon, I. R. H. (2015). *Handbook of behavioural family therapy*. Routledge. https://books.google.co.uk/books?hl=en&lr=&id=9ZhGCgAAQBAJ&oi=fnd&pg=PP1&dq=behavioural+family+therapy&ots=o_mVEItmRm&sig=ZYHbX9rgOCMKos7fiySMCXy3RC0#v=onepage&q=behaviouralfamilytherapy&f=false

Falloon, I. R. H., Boyd, J. L., McGill, C. W., Razani, J., Moss, H. B., & Gilderman, A. M. (1982). Family management in the prevention of exacerbations of schizophrenia. *New England Journal of Medicine*, *306*(24), 1437–1440. https://doi.org/10.1056/NEJM198206173062401

Goh, C., & Agius, M. (2010). The stress-vulnerability model how does stress impact on mental illness at the level of the brain and what are the consequences? *Psychiatria Danubina*, *22*(2), 198–202.

Guest, O., & Martin, A. E. (2021). How computational modeling can force theory building in psychological science. *Perspectives on Psychological Science*, *16*(4), 789–802. https://doi.org/10.1177/1745691620970585

Hayes, L., Hawthorne, G., Farhall, J., O'Hanlon, B., & Harvey, C. (2015). Quality of life and social isolation among caregivers of adults with schizophrenia: Policy and outcomes. *Community Mental Health Journal*, *51*(5), 591–597. https://doi.org/10.1007/s10597-015-9848-6

Hayhurst, H., Cooper, Z., Paykel, E. S., Vearnals, S., & Ramana, R. (1997). Expressed emotion and depression. A longitudinal study. *The British Journal of Psychiatry: The Journal of Mental Science*, *171*, 439–443. https://doi.org/10.1192/bjp.171.5.439

Keeney, B., & Ross, J. (1983). Cybernetics of brief family therapy. *Journal of Marital and Family Therapy*, *9*(4), 375–382.

Kim, E. Y., & Miklowitz, D. J. (2004). Expressed emotion as a predictor of outcome among bipolar patients undergoing family therapy. *Journal of Affective Disorders*, *82*(3), 343–352. https://doi.org/10.1016/j.jad.2004.02.004

Kim, Y., & Chung, C. W. (2014). Factors of prenatal depression by stress-vulnerability and stress-coping models. *Korean Journal of Women Health Nursing*, *20*(1), 38–47. https://doi.org/10.4069/kjwhn.2014.20.1.38

Kuipers, E., Onwumere, J., & Bebbington, P. (2010). Cognitive model of caregiving in psychosis. *British Journal of Psychiatry*, *196*(4), 259–265. https://doi.org/10.1192/bjp.bp.109.070466

Kuipers, L., Leff, J., & Lam, D. (2002). *Family work for schizophrenia: A practical guide* (2nd. ed.) Gaskell.

Lippi, G. (2016). Schizophrenia in a member of the family: Burden, expressed emotion and addressing the needs of the whole family. *The South African Journal of Psychiatry : SAJP : The Journal of the Society of Psychiatrists of South Africa*, *22*(1), 922. https://doi.org/10.4102/sajpsychiatry.v22i1.922

McCann, T. V., Lubman, D. I., & Clark, E. (2011). First-time primary caregivers' experience of caring for young adults with first-episode psychosis. *Schizophrenia Bulletin*, *37*(2), 381–388. https://doi.org/10.1093/schbul/sbp085

McClelland, K. (1994). Perceptual control and social power. *Sociological Perspectives*, *37*(4), 461–496. https://doi.org/10.2307/1389276

McClelland, K. (2022). A fresh look at collective control and conflict. *Paper presented at the 32nd IAPCT Conference and 2022 Annual Meeting*.

McClelland, K., & Mansell, W. (2019). Resolving interpersonal and intrapersonal conflicts : A comparison of the practice of mediation with method-of-levels psychotherapy. *Journal of Integrated Social Sciences*, *9*(1), 1–38.

Onwumere, J., Shiers, D., & Chew-Graham, C. (2016). Understanding the needs of carers of people with psychosis in primary care. *British Journal of General Practice*, 66(649), pp. 400–401). Royal College of General Practitioners. https://doi.org/10.3399/bjgp16X686209

Parker, M. G., Willett, A. B. S., Tyson, S. F., Weightman, A. P., & Mansell, W. (2020). A systematic evaluation of the evidence for perceptual control theory in tracking studies. *Neuroscience & Biobehavioral Reviews, 112*, 616–633. https://doi.org/10.1016/j.neubiorev.2020.02.030

Pharoah, F., Mari, J. J., Rathbone, J., & Wong, W. (2010). Family intervention for schizophrenia. *Cochrane Database of Systematic Reviews, 12*. https://doi.org/10.1002/14651858.CD000088.pub3

Powers, W. T. (1973). *Behavior: The control of perception*. Aldine.

Powers, W. T. (2005). Degrees of freedom in social interactions. In *Living control systems* (p. 300). Benchmark Publications.

Robertson, R. J., Goldstein, D. M., Mermel, M., & Musgrave, M. (1999). Testing the self as a control system: Theoretical and methodological issues. *International Journal of Human-Computer Studies, 50*(6), 571–580. https://doi.org/10.1006/ijhc.1998.0256

Runkel, P. J. (2007). *Casting nets and testing specimens* (2nd ed.). Living Control Systems Publishing.

Schizophrenia Commission. (2012). *The abandoned illness: A report by the Schizophrenia Commission*. www.rethink.org/media/514093/TSC_main_report_14_nov.pdf

Shiraishi, N., & Reilly, J. (2019). Positive and negative impacts of schizophrenia on family caregivers: A systematic review and qualitative meta-summary. *Social Psychiatry and Psychiatric Epidemiology, 54*(3), 277–290. https://doi.org/10.1007/s00127-018-1617-8

Sin, J., Elkes, J., Batchelor, R., Henderson, C., Gillard, S., Woodham, L. A., Chen, T., Aden, A., & Cornelius, V. (2021). Mental health and caregiving experiences of family carers supporting people with psychosis. *Epidemiology and Psychiatric Sciences, 30*, e3. https://doi.org/10.1017/S2045796020001067

Vaughn, C., & Leff, J. (1976). The measurement of expressed emotion in the families of psychiatric patients. *British Journal of Social and Clinical Psychology, 15*(2), 157–165. https://doi.org/10.1111/j.2044-8260.1976.tb00021.x

Willett, A. B. S., Marken, R. S., Parker, M. G., & Mansell, W. (2017). Control blindness: Why people can make incorrect inferences about the intentions of others. *Attention, Perception, and Psychophysics, 79*(3), 841–849. https://doi.org/10.3758/s13414-016-1268-3

Zubin, J., & Spring, B. (1977). Vulnerability: A new view of schizophrenia. *Journal of Abnormal Psychology*, 86, 103–126). American Psychological Association. https://doi.org/10.1037/0021-843X.86.2.103

Chapter 8

Perceptual Control Theory as a Unique Biopsychological Approach to Secondary Mental Healthcare

Introduction

The main focus of this book has been to show how the principles of Perceptual Control Theory (PCT; Powers, 1973, 2005) can guide the transformation of service structures, procedures, and interventions within the secondary care mental health system. We have described a variety of challenges to making these changes and how to address them. A recurring challenge is the widely held view that mental health problems are best addressed through the 'medical model'. This term is typically used to refer treatment that is analogous to many (but by no means all) physical illnesses. In other words, it involves diagnosing the specific illness through identifying specific combinations of symptoms and then treating the illness with a specific agent or procedure. In this chapter, we will use PCT, and contemporary scientific evidence, to argue that the 'medical model' does not follow as a logical consequence of the biology of mental health. Rather, it supports the approach we have proposed in this book that systems should enable patients to exert control and choice, and provide opportunities for problem exploration and the resolution of conflict. We will then compare our PCT approach to alternative 'progressive' approaches within the mental health system, such as open dialogue and trauma-informed care.

The biology of Perceptual Control Theory

Whilst PCT was developed by a control systems engineer to understand the behaviour of living organisms, it was also grounded in biology from the start. The impetus for Powers' insight into control was understanding the workings of the negative feedback control systems that had emulated the homeostatic systems described by biologists such as Walter Cannon and Claude Bernard throughout the previous century (Cziko, 2000). Negative feedback control is a ubiquitous, essential, and fully accepted function of living organisms (Carey et al., 2014; Carpenter, 2004; Cisek, 2019). Importantly, however, only Powers made the explicit insight that it is the perceptual input to a system that is controlled, rather than its output or actions. This insight is critical to the

DOI: 10.4324/9781003041344-8

recommendations we have made in this book. We reviewed the evidence for PCT earlier, but what is the evidence that the control of input, and the principles of PCT that follow – hierarchies, conflict, and reorganisation – are operating within human biology, and are key to understanding mental health?

Powers (1973) described in some detail how the physiology of neurons, and the architecture of the nervous system would implement his model. These proposed properties, which we will not describe in detail here, moulded the way that a handful of neuroscientists have approached their research. Following some earlier published ideas regarding the perceptual hierarchy (e.g., Cools, 1985), Henry Yin at Duke University carried out a series of studies into the neuroscience of behaviour that now form a coherent body of work that supports PCT (Yin, 2020). Yin measured neural activity in animal behaviour during naturalistic, self-initiated actions, rather than the constrained conditions under which animals were usually tested. He found that groups of neurons in specific areas of the brain known to be involved in action control (e.g., the basal ganglia) fired at a rate proportional to variables that were perceived (such as the perception of relative joint position). By compiling the results of studies of this kind, he was able to propose a hierarchy to explain behaviour as controlled perceptual input, at various levels (Yin, 2017). This also allowed him to propose a location of each level within neuroanatomy. Yin and colleagues have now gone on to show the proof-of-concept of this architecture within robotic models of locomotion (Barter & Yin, 2021).

Several other researchers have provided accounts and research programmes that complement Yin's work. Erling Jorgensen has provided a detailed PCT account of the roles of the thalamus as a bank of comparators for negative feedback, the layers of the neocortex in temporal memory, and the occipital cortex in visual perception (Jorgensen, 2020a, 2020b, 2020c). Alex Gomez-Marin and colleagues have also tested the principles of PCT within human and animal experiments, and robotic designs (Gomez-Marin & Ghazanfar, 2019; Matić et al., 2021).

The neuroscience of mental health has not been extensively studied through the lens of PCT. Yet, there is a range of evidence consistent with the principles of control, conflict, and reorganisation (Mansell, 2021). Some of this evidence is critical to how mental health is understood and treated, and can take on new meaning from the perspective of PCT. One classic example is the phenomenon of learned helplessness in animals, which was used as an animal model of depression (Seligman, 1972). In the original studies, animals were subjected to either controllable or uncontrollable electric shocks. Only those animals subjected to the uncontrollable shocks showed what appeared to be the symptoms of 'depression' (characterised by disruptions to 'adaptive responding'). The lack of control in these circumstances appears to be related to a disruption of a brain system known as the HPA-axis – the hypothalamic-pituitary-adrenal axis. Typically, the dysregulation of the HPA is indicated by increased levels of the hormone cortisol in the blood, which is an established indicator for stress and high levels of risk (Resch & Parzer, 2021). Critically, it has been proposed, outside the realms of PCT, that uncontrollable stress requires neural plasticity in order to adapt to stress (Holmes & Wellman, 2009; Huether et al., 1999). In PCT terms this would entail reorganisation of the perceptual hierarchy to restore control.

Not only is lack of control identified as almost synonymous with stress within the wider literature on the neuroscience of mental health, but situations that engender conflict are widely used to examine the brain mechanisms involved (Kirlic et al., 2017). For example, researchers have examined how animals resolve conflict when faced with the decision between the lure of novelty or food that is accompanied by an electric shock, and they have attempted to identify the neural signatures of conflict resolution in humans using a range of experimental paradigms involving, for example, monetary rewards accompanied by mild electric shocks. There is an emerging consensus that conflict resolution is associated with activity in a specific brain network that includes the medial prefrontal cortex, orbital frontal cortex, and the striatum (Kirlic et al., 2017). Whilst there is clearly the potential for both ethical and methodological issues with this body of research, the point to be made is that conflict processing is a well-accepted focus for research relevant to mental health, and even a critical review of the evidence suggests that conflict resolution is a necessary function of the brain.

Biological research on mental health through the PCT lens

It is of huge concern that the Director of the leading medical research council in the USA – the National Institute of Mental Health (NIMH) – Tom Insel has admitted that:

> I spent 13 years at NIMH really pushing on the neuroscience and genetics of mental disorders … I succeeded at getting lots of cool papers by cool scientists at fairly large costs – I think $20 billion – I don't think we moved the needle in reducing suicide, reducing hospitalisations, improving recovery for the tens of millions of people who have mental illness.
>
> (Rogers, 2017, p. 1)

This is a frank admission, but why might such expensive biological research not make an impact? It is not the case that the research studies had null findings. Many of them showed people with certain mental health diagnoses were statistically more likely to share a specific gene. Also, it is not simply the case that the research was based on a purely medical, diagnostic model. For example, in recent years there has been a wealth of research identifying genes that may raise vulnerability across diagnostic categories (e.g., Allegrini et al., 2020), and studies of brain mechanisms that are transdiagnostic (e.g., Dadds & Frick, 2019).

Rather, what seems to be missing is the link between the science and 'improving recovery'. Classically, the goal is to identify the so-called 'biomarkers' of a specific brain mechanism and 'treat' it directly. Historically, this was the justification for drastic and debilitating surgical operations of psychiatric patients such as frontal leucotomies. At present, it may be used to justify certain pharmaceutical interventions, or more recently, transcranial magnetic stimulation (TMS) to specific locations of the brain. Rather than critique the validity, costs, and benefits of such interventions here, they serve as a contrast to the PCT explanation of the role of biology within a theoretical framework that is utilised for mental health interventions.

One example is the biology of bipolar disorder. One of the most longstanding and prevalent views is that bipolar disorder results from an overactive 'reward' system of the brain (e.g., Satterthwaite et al., 2015). In fact, this account stretches to people who are described as 'hypomania-prone' (Mason et al., 2012), that is people who don't have a diagnosis of bipolar disorder and who report statements such as 'At social gatherings, I am usually the "life of the party"'. Whilst people who report these kinds of statements are more likely to be diagnosed with bipolar disorder later in life, the majority of them are not. So, what we have here is an individual difference in the degree to which people strive for success, often in a way that is urgent or impulsive. The term 'positive urgency' has been used to describe a tendency to act impulsively in the context of positive affective states (Johnson et al., 2016).

Not only does the individual difference in so-called 'positive urgency' raise vulnerability for a broad range of mental health problems (i.e., it is transdiagnostic), but the available neuroanatomical evidence indicates that 'the real culprit may be the loss of control over high-emotion states generally, rather than positive or negative emotion specifically' (Johnson et al., 2020, p. 10). Thus, we return to the fundamental issue of control, and how to help our patients maintain it in the short and long term, despite the 'emotional challenges' that they may experience. One of the most critical challenges to the emotional state of any individual is what is commonly described in the psychological literature as 'trauma'. Psychological trauma is partly defined by the experience of helplessness, which is lack of control, as mentioned earlier, and the biological signatures of psychological trauma during childhood overlap with those often regarded as genetic in origin (Read et al., 2001). Thus, again, the biology of mental health points back to issues with control.

The work on emotion regulation in bipolar disorder ends up treading the same path as many other research programmes on specific mental health problems. The central mechanism identified by these neurocognitive studies can go by various terms including 'cognitive control', 'effortful control', 'attentional control', and 'cognitive flexibility'. Each of these terms has a largely overlapping, and somewhat distinct, definition, but none of them is constructed from a working model of control itself, which comes from the application of control engineering by Powers through PCT. Those using these terms implicitly acknowledge that the cognitive control process needs to resolve conflict, but conflict in this context means 'response conflict' – what behaviour to carry out in a specific situation – as is the case performing activities such as the Stroop task (Cohen et al., 1990). The role of cognitive control, from this perspective, is typically to select a behavioural response. In contrast, within PCT, the nervous system is understood to be a hierarchical system that controls its inputs; the most fundamental conflict is at the highest levels in the hierarchy, and the resolution of this conflict requires shifting and sustaining attention to the source of the conflict to allow the trial-and-error discovery of a higher-level perception that, when controlled, re-establishes control. Indeed, within what is elsewhere interpreted as psychological trauma, this remains the focus of the Method of Levels (MOL), the PCT-informed psychological intervention described in Chapter 4 (Carey et al., 2014).

A critical aspect of this book is our contention that the active process of change is the shifting and focusing of awareness to the level above two systems in perceptual conflict. One way to test for evidence of this process is to code the language used by people when they attempt to describe a problem. The text can be analysed for the presence of terms that indicate the person is aware of conflicting goals – for example 'being in two minds' or 'one part of me wants X and another part of me wants Y'. We called this goal conflict awareness. Two studies have found that people who report being less distressed about their problems after a psychological intervention are those who use more of this kind of language (Gaffney et al., 2014; Kelly et al., 2012). We have also developed a questionnaire that allows people to report on how they face problems, and it includes items that tap into goal conflict awareness such as 'When I have a problem it often feels like there are two sides of me wanting different things'. The scale also attempts to assess the experience of having a problem that is resolved by reorganisation, such as 'Once I've worked through a difficult time it feels like something has just shifted into place'. In a number of studies of MOL, scores on this scale, known as the Reorganisation of Conflict Scale, tend to reduce over the course of the intervention (Churchman et al., 2021; Griffiths et al., 2019). One of the research methods with greatest potential to study the process of goal conflict reorganisation is computational modelling, and a recent review summarises this approach (Mansell, 2020).

Interestingly, it is possible to reach the same conclusions regarding goal conflict awareness and tolerance of reorganisation by exploring the role of medication in treating mental health problems. Take bipolar disorder again. First to note is that almost every kind of psychotropic medication has been used as a 'treatment': mood stabilisers, antidepressants, anticonvulsants, antipsychotics, and anxiolytics. This illustrates the lack of a focused mechanism for pharmacological treatments. Second, in contrast, there is evidence that medication reduces the risk of what is described as 'relapse' in many people, and with it many of the harmful consequences (Geddes et al., 2004). A large minority of patients, however, are still judged to have experienced a relapse within two years, even when blood samples indicate they are keeping to their medication regime (Solomon et al., 1997). Taking these points together, it is clear that for any one individual, whether or not to take medication to reduce relapse, and which medication to take, is not certain from the diagnosis alone. There is a fundamental conflict between taking medication to try to prevent a dangerous relapse (even though this is not in any way guaranteed), versus reducing medication in order to limit side effects and potentially reduce drug-dependence and improve recovery.

A case series of MOL in secondary care has indicated that attitudes towards medication can be a helpful focus for some patients, helping them to make a balanced decision (Dicks, 2019). Indeed, there is now increasing evidence that drugs, such as psychedelics, that have the opposite effect to traditional medication on emotional experience – enhancing it, rather than suppressing it – may be effective in supporting the benefits of psychological therapy (Perkins et al., 2021). Again, MOL is being used in this context (Tai et al., 2021). Moreover, the proposal is that psychedelic drugs may help to reduce habitual attempts at controlling emotional experiences, thereby allowing people to sustain awareness for longer on conflicted control systems, supporting reorganisation (Tai et al., 2021). According to PCT, it is critical that this is done in a safe environment in which the patient feels in control. In many ways, people's accounts of using psychedelic drugs are similar to first-person reports of experiencing psychosis. A PCT-informed service model involves providing the support and attention that patients need to explore distressing experiences of psychosis, and, if and when they want to, use this as a means to support personal recovery. For many patients, this supportive, open, curious environment is critical. For example, one expert through lived experience provided an account of a mental health nurse who supported him to write down his stream of thoughts continuously, and viewing them afterwards helped him to generate a theory of his own recovery (Tolton, 2006).

PCT as a biopsychosocial framework versus alternative contemporary approaches

The principles of PCT make it clearly distinct from other contemporary approaches to secondary mental healthcare interventions, even though there are some notable overlaps. In this section, we will draw out some of these overlaps and distinctions.

Whilst we have contrasted PCT interventions with CBT in various sections of the book, we have made less explicit comparison with contemporary 'process-focused' interventions. One advance has been to deliver highly focused interventions on a specific process, such as anxious avoidance, worry, low self-esteem, or insomnia (D. Freeman et al., 2019b). Whilst the initial results are promising, there are also some limitations. First, the specific problems would need to be identified, and training and provision for separate treatment modules provided. Second, it still leaves the question of who decides upon the treatment focus where multiple treatment targets are identified, or where none are identified. By default, a PCT approach would leave this decision to the patient. Third, there are reasons to believe that these processes indicate more fundamental issues or conflicts to resolve. Many of these potential 'treatment targets' in psychosis are also symptoms experienced by patients with PTSD. Yet, the recommended psychological treatment is to address the processing of the underlying trauma memory (Ehlers & Wild, 2015). For example, case studies have shown that MOL in people reporting insomnia has improved sleep, and reduced anxiety and depression, even when none of these was the direct problem of choice covered during the therapy (Grzegrzolka et al., 2019).

Another field of process-focused therapy includes 'third wave' approaches such as compassion-focused therapy, acceptance and commitment therapy (ACT), and mindfulness training (Tai & Turkington, 2009). Again, these interventions are promising in their results. Moreover, there are some conceptual similarities with PCT. For example, mindfulness training may help to enhance the control over awareness and the curious, accepting stance cultivated in MOL (Mansell, 2009), and ACT involves helping patients to access and articulate higher level goals – values – that provide a new perspective on their difficulties. A key difference in therapeutic practice, however, comes from the principles of PCT. For example, the principles of PCT can form the basis even for a simple discussion with a patient about their current problems – relationships with staff members, medication, preference for where to stay on a ward. The basis is that the patient leads the topic and is helped to talk openly and freely where they wish to. The practitioner follows what they are saying carefully, asking questions for clarification, and occasionally helping direct attention to any background thoughts about the issue. Where there is no obvious requirement to have a mindful training exercise, or to pinpoint the patient's underlying values, then this is not part of the conversation. In this way, we would propose that a PCT intervention blends seamlessly into everyday interactions and imbues the principles of the service and its staff.

There are potentially powerful initiatives that do attempt to shift the ethos of mental health services as a whole, and again they share some similarities with PCT-informed care. For example, there is an increasing awareness that services should be trauma-informed (e.g., Molloy et al., 2020). Whilst this is being most effectively implemented within child services, the implications for adult mental health are making it a priority. Given what we covered earlier regarding the nature of trauma being one of lack of control experienced as helplessness, awareness of trauma is clearly also critical to PCT-informed services. Yet the emphasis is very different. Whilst the evidence indicates that most secondary care patients have experienced childhood trauma, that does not imply that they will want to disclose and describe their trauma to a clinician. Of course, it also does not apply that the potential history of trauma should be ignored or minimised by the clinician. If the clinician does not feel ready or sufficiently experienced to discuss the topic proposed by the patient, then this is an issue for the service itself to address (not the patient), potentially by drawing upon the necessary expertise within the service. The PCT-informed practitioner works with whatever problem the patient wishes to discuss, and this includes trauma, as and when the patient chooses to talk about it. An additional advantage of a PCT-informed service is that the patient does not need to share the details of the trauma in order to work on it in the session. As long as they can hold some feature of their experience in mind and explore it, they do not need to divulge details such as specific dates, individuals concerned, or locations. For some patients this can be very empowering and free them from fears of being judged or accused.

Another issue to consider is who is best placed to define past experiences as 'traumatic'. Developing a general definition of trauma and finding reliable and valid methods of measurement has been challenging (Weathers & Keane, 2007). A variety of outcome measures have been developed for this purpose (Brewin, 2005), and attempts have been made to parse traumatic events into 'direct' and 'indirect' types (May & Wisco, 2016). The DSM-5 defines trauma as occurring in the context of 'actual or threatened death, serious injury, or sexual violence' (APA, 2013, p. 271), excluding other forms of stressful life event (Pai et al., 2017). In contrast to these approaches, the patient-perspective approach (Carey, 2017), informed by PCT, means that the person reporting the distressing problem can decide whether the term 'trauma' accurately describes their past experiences.

In terms of the therapy itself, a PCT service would offer MOL to patients with a history of trauma. This makes sense – trauma is transdiagnostic and pervasive – limiting MOL to patients without trauma would contradict this. More importantly, the conflict around trauma is key (Carey et al., 2014). On an immediate level this is often the conflict over whether to allow re-experiencing of traumatic intrusive memories, or whether to try to block them out in various ways – mental effort, distraction, medication, drink, and drugs. On a higher level, this conflict is more fundamental. For example, one patient wanted to forget her assault had ever happened so she could get on with her life and stay close to her family who were friends of her attacker. Yet she also wanted justice and she wanted to make sure the perpetrator did not attack any other young women. To do this, she would have to give a detailed account of the trauma to the police – the exact opposition from suppressing it. For this patient, MOL allowed her to talk about and tolerate this conflict over time and eventually, when the perpetrator pleaded guilty in court and went to prison, both goals were achieved – her family were supportive, and justice and safety were ensured.

The spirit of PCT-informed care is to facilitate awareness and open expression of whatever the patients regard as important to them. Trauma may often be one of these issues. The initiative of Open Dialogue is another principle-based approach to services, and it resonates with some aspects of PCT (A. Freeman et al., 2019a). This approach provides patients, families, and services with a safe space to make transparent decisions and to put their experiences in words. It locates problems across networks of individuals rather than within one person, and it explores how social interactions shape mental health problems. Theoretically, the approach integrates systemic family therapy, some psychodynamic principles, and social constructionism. Without going into too much detail, some obvious differences are evident. First, PCT is a single theoretical framework that operates according to the same principles at the social, psychological, and biological level. Second, this allows it to potentially interface between the cultural, social, psychological, and biological domains as we have described here, rather than to prioritise the socially constructed nature of reality. Third, and relatedly, whilst a mental health problem can be a feature of a network of controlling agents (or, put more simply: a group of people), it is also a feature of conflict within the individual. As such, opportunities should be provided for individual patients to make the changes and insights they require. Ultimately, our vision is of a society in which mental health problems are understood to be issues of control and conflict, to be remedied by awareness and reorganisation. In a society that understood mental health difficulties in this way, effective peer support would be the norm, and medical services would only be needed where prevention and promotion were unsuccessful, such as in the fields of dental care or emergency medicine.

Summary

Over the course of this book, we have sought to describe how PCT might be applied to the design and delivery of secondary mental healthcare, with the aim of making these services more helpful for the people who use them. We have argued that the serious and wide-ranging problems described by patients with experience of accessing care from these services could be addressed by shifting to a model of patient-perspective mental healthcare that was informed by the principles of PCT.

As they are currently designed, mental health services are often experienced as coercive, inflexible, and insufficiently focused on addressing the problems that are prioritised by patients. They also do not appear to be informed by a set of coherent theoretical principles.

PCT offers a radically different way to think about the nature of mental health problems. It also offers novel solutions for how we might go about addressing these problems to help people lead the lives that they want to. From a PCT perspective, the problem that needs to be addressed by mental health services is disrupted control – people experience distress when they are unable to control important aspects of their lives satisfactorily. Mental health services need to be designed to help people maintain or regain control over those things that they value (in PCT terms, to act as part of an individual's feedback function, rather than as a disturbance).

Research into the design of mental health services and approaches that are informed by PCT is still in its early stages. Throughout this book, however, we have described the progress made so far, and offered some suggestions for possible areas of future research in this area. We hope that the ideas in this book will have sparked your interest in the theory and conveyed a sense of how PCT might address some of the profound and wide-spread problems that exist with mental health services as they are currently delivered.

References

Allegrini, A. G., Cheesman, R., Rimfeld, K., Selzam, S., Pingault, J.-B., Eley, T. C., & Plomin, R. (2020). The p factor: Genetic analyses support a general dimension of psychopathology in childhood and adolescence. *Journal of Child Psychology and Psychiatry, and Allied Disciplines*, *61*(1), 30–39. https://doi.org/10.1111/jcpp.13113

American Psychological Association. (2013). *Diagnostic and statistical manual of mental disorders (5th edition)*. American Psychological Association. https://dsm.psychiatryonline.org/doi/book/10.1176/appi.books.9780890425596

Barter, J. W., & Yin, H. H. (2021). Achieving natural behavior in a robot using neurally inspired hierarchical perceptual control. *IScience*, *24*(9), 102948. https://doi.org/10.1016/j.isci.2021.102948

Brewin, C. R. (2005). Risk factor effect sizes in PTSD: What this means for intervention. *Journal of Trauma & Dissociation*, *6*(2), 123–130. https://doi.org/10.1300/J229v06n02_11

Carey, T. A. (2017). *Patient-perspective care: A new paradigm for health systems and services* (1st ed.). Routledge.

Carey, T. A., Mansell, W., Tai, S. J., & Turkington, D. (2014). Conflicted control systems: The neural architecture of trauma. *The Lancet Psychiatry*, *1*(4), 316–318. https://doi.org/10.1016/S2215-0366(14)70306-2

Carpenter, R. H. S. (2004). Homeostasis: A plea for a unified approach. *Advances in Physiology Education*, *28*(4), 180–187. https://doi.org/10.1152/advan.00012.2004

Churchman, A., Mansell, W., & Tai, S. (2021). A process-focused case series of a school-based intervention aimed at giving young people choice and control over their attendance and their goals in therapy. *British Journal of Guidance & Counselling*, *49*(4), 565–586. https://doi.org/10.1080/03069885.2020.1815650

Cisek, P. (2019). Resynthesizing behavior through phylogenetic refinement. *Attention, Perception, & Psychophysics*, *81*(7), 2265–2287. https://doi.org/10.3758/s13414-019-01760-1

Cohen, J. D., Dunbar, K., & McClelland, J. L. (1990). On the control of automatic processes: A parallel distributed processing account of the Stroop effect. *Psychological Review*, *97*, 332–361). American Psychological Association. https://doi.org/10.1037/0033-295X.97.3.332

Cools, A. R. (1985). *Brain and behavior: Hierarchy of feedback systems and control of input BT – perspectives in ethology: Volume 6 Mechanisms* (P. P. G. Bateson & P. H. Klopfer (Eds.); pp. 109–168). Springer US. https://doi.org/10.1007/978-1-4757-0232-3_5

Cziko, G. A. (2000). *The things we do: Using the lessons of Bernard and Darwin to understand the what, how, and why of our behavior*. MIT Press.

Dadds, M. R., & Frick, P. J. (2019). Toward a transdiagnostic model of common and unique processes leading to the major disorders of childhood: The REAL model of attention, responsiveness and learning. *Behaviour Research and Therapy*, *119*, 103410. https://doi.org/10.1016/j.brat.2019.103410

Dicks, R. E. (2019). *Interventions to facilitate service user decisions around medication use for mental health difficulties*. Doctoral thesis submitted to University of Manchester.

Ehlers, A., & Wild, J. (2015). Cognitive therapy for PTSD: Updating memories and meanings of trauma. In U. Schnyder & M. Cloitre (Eds.), *Evidence based treatments for trauma-related psychological disorders: A practical guide for clinicians* (pp. 161–187). Springer International Publishing/Springer Nature. https://doi.org/10.1007/978-3-319-07109-1_9

Freeman, A. M., Tribe, R. H., Stott, J. C. H., & Pilling, S. (2019a). Open dialogue: A review of the evidence. *Psychiatric Services (Washington, D.C.)*, *70*(1), 46–59. https://doi.org/10.1176/appi.ps.201800236

Freeman, D., Taylor, K. M., Molodynski, A., & Waite, F. (2019b). Treatable clinical intervention targets for patients with schizophrenia. *Schizophrenia Research*, *211*, 44–50. https://doi.org/10.1016/j.schres.2019.07.016

Gaffney, H., Mansell, W., Edwards, R., & Wright, J. (2014). Manage Your Life Online (MYLO): A pilot trial of a conversational computer-based intervention for problem solving in a student sample. *Behavioural and Cognitive Psychotherapy*, *42*(6), 731–746. https://doi.org/10.1017/S135246581300060X

Geddes, J. R., Burgess, S., Hawton, K., Jamison, K., & Goodwin, G. M. (2004). Long-term lithium therapy for bipolar disorder: Systematic review and meta-analysis of randomized controlled trials. *The American Journal of Psychiatry*, *161*(2), 217–222. https://doi.org/10.1176/appi.ajp.161.2.217

Gomez-Marin, A., & Ghazanfar, A. A. (2019). The life of behavior. *Neuron*, *104*(1), 25–36. https://doi.org/10.1016/j.neuron.2019.09.017

Griffiths, R., Mansell, W., Carey, T. A., Edge, D., Emsley, R., & Tai, S. J. (2019). Method of levels therapy for first-episode psychosis: The feasibility randomized controlled Next Level trial. *Journal of Clinical Psychology*, *75*(10), 1756–1769. https://doi.org/10.1002/jclp.22820

Grzegrzolka, J., McEvoy, P., & Mansell, W. (2019). Use of the Method of Levels therapy as a low-intensity intervention to work with people experiencing sleep difficulties. *Journal of Cognitive Psychotherapy*, *33*(2), 140–156. https://doi.org/10.1891/0889-8391.33.2.140

Holmes, A., & Wellman, C. L. (2009). Stress-induced prefrontal reorganization and executive dysfunction in rodents. *Neuroscience and Biobehavioral Reviews*, *33*(6), 773–783. https://doi.org/10.1016/j.neubiorev.2008.11.005

Huether, G., Doering, S., Rüger, U., Rüther, E., & Schüssler, G. (1999). The stress-reaction process and the adaptive modification and reorganization of neuronal networks. *Psychiatry Research*, *87*(1), 83–95. https://doi.org/10.1016/s0165-1781(99)00044-x

Johnson, S. L., Elliott, M. V., & Carver, C. S. (2020). Impulsive responses to positive and negative emotions: Parallel neurocognitive correlates and their implications. *Biological Psychiatry*, *87*(4), 338–349. https://doi.org/10.1016/j.biopsych.2019.08.018

Johnson, S. L., Tharp, J. A., Peckham, A. D., Sanchez, A. H., & Carver, C. S. (2016). Positive urgency is related to difficulty inhibiting prepotent responses. *Emotion (Washington, D.C.)*, *16*(5), 750–759. https://doi.org/10.1037/emo0000182

Jorgensen, E. O. (2020a). *Chapter 17 – How the brain gets a roaring campfire: Structuring for perceptual results* (W. B. T.–T. I. H. of P. C. T. Mansell (Ed.); p. e1.1–e1.51). Academic Press. https://doi.org/10.1016/B978-0-12-818948-1.00017-4

Jorgensen, E. O. (2020b). *Chapter 18 – How the brain gets a roaring campfire: Input and output functions* (W. B. T.–T. I. H. of P. C. T. Mansell (Ed.); p. e2.1–e2.73). Academic Press. https://doi.org/10.1016/B978-0-12-818948-1.00018-6

Jorgensen, E. O. (2020c). *Chapter 19 – How the brain gets a roaring campfire: Thalamus through a PCT microscope* (W. B. T.–T. I. H. of P. C. T. Mansell (Ed.); p. e3.1–e3.42). Academic Press. https://doi.org/10.1016/B978-0-12-818948-1.00019-8

Kelly, R. E., Wood, A. M., Shearman, K., Phillips, S., & Mansell, W. (2012). Encouraging acceptance of ambivalence using the expressive writing paradigm. *Psychology and Psychotherapy*, *85*(2), 220–228. https://doi.org/10.1111/j.2044-8341.2011.02023.x

Kirlic, N., Young, J., & Aupperle, R. L. (2017). Animal to human translational paradigms relevant for approach avoidance conflict decision making. *Behaviour Research and Therapy*, *96*, 14–29. https://doi.org/10.1016/j.brat.2017.04.010

Mansell, W. (2009). Perceptual Control Theory as an integrative framework and Method of Levels as a cognitive therapy: What are the pros and cons? *The Cognitive Behaviour Therapist*, *2*(2001), 178. https://doi.org/10.1017/S1754470X08000093

Mansell, W. (2020). – Ten vital elements of perceptual control theory, tracing the pathway from implicit influence to scientific advance, *The International Handbook of Perceptual Control Theory*, W. Mansell (Ed.); pp. 585–629). Academic Press. https://doi.org/10.1016/B978-0-12-818948-1.00016-2

Mansell, W. (2021). The perceptual control model of psychopathology. *Current Opinion in Psychology*, *41*, 15–20. https://doi.org/10.1016/j.copsyc.2021.01.008

Mason, L., O'Sullivan, N., Bentall, R. P., & El-Deredy, W. (2012). Better than I thought: Positive evaluation bias in hypomania. *PloS One*, *7*(10), e47754. https://doi.org/10.1371/journal.pone.0047754

Matić, A., Valerjev, P., & Gomez-Marin, A. (2021). Hierarchical control of visually-guided movements in a 3D-printed robot arm. *Frontiers in Neurorobotics*, *15*. www.frontiersin.org/articles/10.3389/fnbot.2021.755723

May, C. L., & Wisco, B. E. (2016). Defining trauma: How level of exposure and proximity affect risk for posttraumatic stress disorder. *Psychological Trauma: Theory, Research, Practice and Policy*, *8*(2), 233–240. https://doi.org/10.1037/tra0000077

Molloy, L., Fields, L., Trostian, B., & Kinghorn, G. (2020). Trauma-informed care for people presenting to the emergency department with mental health issues. *Emergency Nurse: The Journal of the RCN Accident and Emergency Nursing Association*, *28*(2), 30–35. https://doi.org/10.7748/en.2020.e1990

Pai, A., Suris, A. M., & North, C. S. (2017). Posttraumatic stress disorder in the DSM-5: Controversy, change, and conceptual considerations. *Behavioral Sciences (Basel, Switzerland)*, *7*(1). https://doi.org/10.3390/bs7010007

Perkins, D., Sarris, J., Rossell, S., Bonomo, Y., Forbes, D., Davey, C., Hoyer, D., Loo, C., Murray, G., Hood, S., Schubert, V., Galvão-Coelho, N. L., O'Donnell, M., Carter, O., Liknaitzky, P., Williams, M., Siskind, D., Penington, D., Berk, M., & Castle, D. (2021). Medicinal psychedelics for mental health and addiction: Advancing research of an emerging paradigm. *The Australian and New Zealand Journal of Psychiatry*, *55*(12), 1127–1133. https://doi.org/10.1177/0004867421998785

Powers, W. T. (1973). *Behavior: The control of perception*. Aldine.

Powers, W. T. (2005). *Behavior: The control of perception* (2nd ed.). Benchmark Publications.

Read, J., Perry, B. D., Moskowitz, A., & Connolly, J. (2001). The contribution of early traumatic events to schizophrenia in some patients: a traumagenic neurodevelopmental model. *Psychiatry*, *64*(4), 319–345. https://doi.org/10.1521/psyc.64.4.319.18602

Resch, F., & Parzer, P. (2021). *Adolescent risk behavior and self-regulation* (1st ed.). Springer Cham.

Rogers, A. (2017, May). Star neuroscientist Tom Insel leaves the Google-spawned verily for … a startup? *Wired.* www.wired.com/2017/05/star-neuroscientist-tom-insel-leaves-google-spawned-verily-startup/?mbid=social_fb_onsiteshare

Satterthwaite, T. D., Kable, J. W., Vandekar, L., Katchmar, N., Bassett, D. S., Baldassano, C. F., Ruparel, K., Elliott, M. A., Sheline, Y. I., Gur, R. C., Gur, R. E., Davatzikos, C., Leibenluft, E., Thase, M. E., & Wolf, D. H. (2015). Common and dissociable dysfunction of the reward system in bipolar and unipolar depression. *Neuropsychopharmacology: Official Publication of the American College of Neuropsychopharmacology*, *40*(9), 2258–2268. https://doi.org/10.1038/npp.2015.75

Seligman, M. E. P. (1972). Learned helplessness. *Annual Review of Medicine*, *23*(1), 407–412. https://doi.org/10.1146/annurev.me.23.020172.002203

Solomon, D. A., Ryan, C. E., Keitner, G. I., Miller, I. W., Shea, M. T., Kazim, A., & Keller, M. B. (1997). A pilot study of lithium carbonate plus divalproex sodium for the continuation and maintenance treatment of patients with bipolar I disorder. *The Journal of Clinical Psychiatry*, *58*(3), 95–99. https://doi.org/10.4088/jcp.v58n0301

Tai, S. J., Nielson, E. M., Lennard-Jones, M., Johanna Ajantaival, R. L., Winzer, R., Richards, W. A., Reinholdt, F., Richards, B. D., Gasser, P., & Malievskaia, E. (2021). Development and evaluation of a therapist training program for psilocybin therapy for treatment-resistant depression in clinical research. *Frontiers in Psychiatry*, *12*(February), 1–9. https://doi.org/10.3389/fpsyt.2021.586682

Tai, S., & Turkington, D. (2009). The evolution of cognitive behavior therapy for schizophrenia: Current practice and recent developments. *Schizophrenia Bulletin*, *35*(5), 865–873. https://doi.org/10.1093/schbul/sbp080

Tolton, J. C. (2006). Rogue psychotic mindset … the cerebral seat of delusive misconception? *Behavioural and Cognitive Psychotherapy*, *34*(4), 487–490. https://doi.org10.1017/S1352465806002955

Weathers, F. W., & Keane, T. M. (2007). The criterion a problem revisited: Controversies and challenges in defining and measuring psychological trauma. *Journal of Traumatic Stress*, *20*(2), 107–121. https://doi.org/10.1002/jts.20210

Yin, H. (2020). *The crisis in neuroscience* (W. B. T.–T. I. H. of P. C. T. Mansell (Ed.); pp. 23–48). Academic Press. https://doi.org/10.1016/B978-0-12-818948-1.00003-4

Yin, H. H. (2017). The basal ganglia in action. *The Neuroscientist: A Review Journal Bringing Neurobiology, Neurology and Psychiatry*, *23*(3), 299–313. https://doi.org/10.1177/1073858416654115

Index

Pages in *italics* refer to figures.